Chef Scenarios

Case Studies, Case Histories, and Narratives on Teaching, and Leadership in Kitchen Classrooms and in Industry

Sharon D. Hartnett, Ph.D.
Seattle Pacific University

Claudette Lévesque
Johnson & Wales University

Contributors: *Laird Livingston*
Ron Koetter

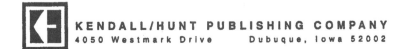
KENDALL/HUNT PUBLISHING COMPANY
4050 Westmark Drive   Dubuque, Iowa 52002

Cover photo courtesy of Charlie Trotter's and photographer, Paul Elledge.

Amy Pleasant
Amy is a freelance illustrator at the Art Institute of Seattle. She has published work for various educational curriculum materials. She is involved in painting and printmaking and has developed a line of greeting cards from her block prints. She also teaches sixth grade for the Shoreline School District and resides in Seattle, Washington.

Dedication

For Fr. John F. Hurley, S.J.

&

Rev. Monsignor Edmond R. Lévesque

Contents

Foreword

For more than 30 years of my life, I have been immersed in the culinary world. As a student, a faculty member, department chairperson, director, dean, and administrator, I have always wondered why so many talented chefs struggle in an attempt to share their vast knowledge and creativity with their students. Their talents are fruitless if they are unable to share their skills with others who are willing and eager to learn.

Now, as President of the Providence Campus of Johnson & Wales University, the largest Culinary Institution in the world, it is my mission to ensure that our faculty are able to teach and inspire our students to become great chefs. What Dr. Sharon Hartnett and Dr. Claudette Lévesque have finally given us is a unique, much needed venue to help in this quest: a textbook to teach chefs how to teach.

The case studies, histories, questions, and narratives are insightful, unique, and interesting. I found myself reading the book in one sitting, much like one would savor a fine meal. So please sit back, take in everything this book has to offer, and utilize it to inspire others. This resource will enable all culinarians involved in education to be more effective teachers. Ultimately, students will benefit from more progressive instruction and innovative learning techniques and our goal of cultivating successful and effective culinary educators will be achieved.

John J. Bowen '77
President—Providence Campus
Johnson & Wales University
September, 2001

Introduction

Thousands who are trained as chefs will at one time or another find themselves in a teaching environment. This book is written in response to the numerous requests that we received from individuals who work in the college systems. These chef educators voiced their concerns about teaching culinary art skills in an academic environment without having had any prior classroom experience. In an attempt to become effective educators, they sought assistance in developing instructional strategies, leadership skills, and management techniques.

Managing people, resources, ideas, facilities, and budgets are problems that are common to chefs in academe and industry alike. The case studies, case histories, and narratives are therefore derived from both sectors. These resources are designed for use by both industry and classroom chefs to encourage discussion and a sharing of ideas. Part 1 of *Chef Scenarios* deals with Teaching Strategies, Teacher Burnout, and Classroom Management, and is written from the perspective of chef educators. The information provided here can assist chefs and students to reflect on what it takes to successfully assume the career of chef/educator. Situations that might occur in the classroom and topics such as teacher morale and communicating with students, colleagues, and administrators are all examined.

Part II—Leadership, Management, and Organizational Theory is written from the perspective of chefs in industry. This section addresses topics such as providing quality guest service, communicating with employees, and managing a budget while creating a quality product. Problems in balancing both a job and family life are also looked at.

Acknowledgments

A sincere thank you to the chefs at Spokane Community College who invited us into their world of culinary arts to experience their craft. Their interest in better serving students presented us the opportunity to write this book. To Brian Shafar, Susan Mourcade, Colletta Young, Edward Orsborn, Vanessa Hermes, Frank Kline, and Susan Franklin, my gratitude.

Our deepest appreciation also goes out to Linda Salisbury, Pam Ashford, Charlotte Akin, Joan Kuhn, Sahron Stampalia, and Bradley Ware for believing in our ability to complete this project.

PART 1

Teaching Strategies, Teacher Burnout, and Classroom Management

EXPERIENCES OF CHEF EDUCATORS

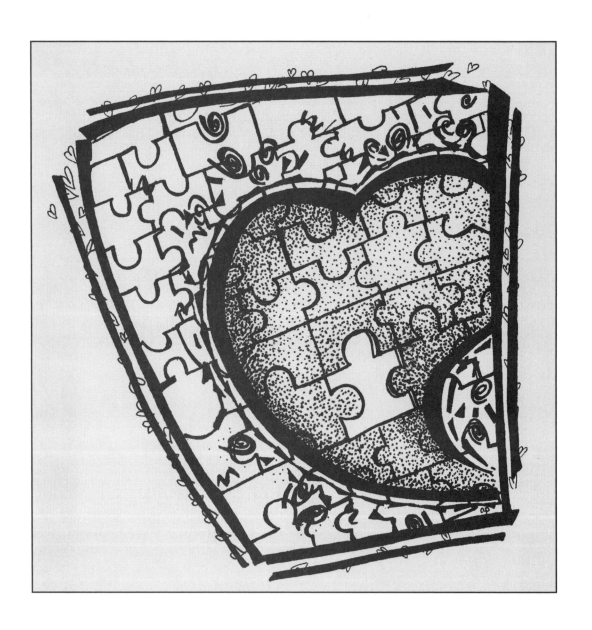

It Takes Courage to Have Ambition
Chef J. Bosich

Without Ambition, People Get Immobilized

Without ambition people become complacent. Although ambition can be defined in many ways, five key words come into the working definition of ambition: desire, drive, dreams, dedication, and determination. Are you afraid to read on? Don't be. Fearing a challenge when it comes one's way is common, as is procrastination in dealing with the task.

When It Gets to Be a Chore, People Avoid It

The key to success is passion. Only true desire to achieve a goal will make it feasible. I know that anything that I have ever enjoyed in life demanded passion. That is what it comes down to for me. A gentleman who was helping to lay out new equipment that had just been delivered to my kitchen asked what he would have to do to become a chef. "Do you just have to shell out $30,000?" he asked. I answered that" $30,000 is a start, but that passion and desire are needed to achieve such a goal." He was speechless and I believe that he decided to keep his day job. It takes years of practice to become a competent chef. Long hours in the kitchen and an enjoyment of the work are integral.

What Does Passion Look Like?

Passion is enthusiasm, energy, and desire. Enthusiasm is the motivator, energy is needed to carry on the mission, and desire is necessary to achieve success. Inspiring students is not a job for everyone. To help students find a place in our business, in which they can achieve success, takes time, energy, patience, and above all, a passion for the food industry.

Passion is not relative to age, background, or demographics. It is a conscious choice to think in a particular way. Career changes occur because there is a passion for change in individuals who are sick and tired of being sick and tired.

But Chef, Some People Don't Want to Learn

I constantly try to encourage my staff to look for a small spark within those whom they teach. I know that student behavior can sometimes "drag instructors down". Many students are financially pressed, they may have problems at home, or come through our doors with a chip on the shoulder. It is our job to confront those issues and to motivate them to succeed. A motto that I try to remember daily is that "I am responsible for my day." This motto places personal responsibility on every individual involved in the learning process. It also provides a framework from which to operate. When instructors at our college have problems with student absenteeism or tardiness, they remind students of this slogan and ask them to also remember why they are with us.

We were created to learn. If students do not want to learn, perhaps they are in the wrong field. Responsibility for being on time, coming to class prepared, and having enthusiasm are all pieces of the puzzle. Although individuals sometimes have every good intention about becoming a chef, they may need direction in reaching their goals. Helping them to build a good work ethic is part of this process. Those who will succeed in the food industry must have the passion and the persistence to spend long hours in the kitchen every day.

Having a Dream Creates Balance

A career in the food industry is ultra-consuming. The demand for production is at times grueling. Yet, I find it a rewarding job that I truly love to do. When I first began to work in industry I found myself getting so wrapped up in my job that I was missing things that were really important in life. I missed friends' weddings, birthdays, and even Mother's Day. One day I realized that I didn't have a life and that I was caught up in a cycle, working from 6 in the morning until 8 o'clock at night, day after day. I knew that I had to force myself to schedule some time off—time that was going to be just for me. If I didn't do this I would soon experience "burnout." I know that I am not alone when I say that it is difficult to remember to save time for yourself. One day a good friend of mine said, "Jill, that palm pilot of yours schedules time for everyone but you." He could see that I looked exhausted. At that point, I decided to take time to go to church, attend special occasions with friends, to work out at the gym, or to go to a movie. This time that I provided myself allowed me to relax and reflect, and to return to work with much more to offer people with whom I work.

Chefs naturally focus on others, so it is a complete shift in thinking to tend to personal needs and priorities, but it is important! This morning I cooked fresh asparagus and drizzled olive oil on them (oil that I had purchased in Italy during a recent trip). I now get up every day and make a lunch that I bring to work. I spend a part of each Sunday preparing meals that I merely have to heat during my hectic work week. When I get home, I can enjoy a quality meal in a few short minutes. I feel better psychologically and physically because of the changes that I've made. When a chef is too tired to cook at home, this is an indication that burnout is close at hand. It is important for a chef to enjoy food away from work as well.

Why It is so Hard to Learn to Say, No?

Setting boundaries is not initially an easy task, but ultimately it does pay big dividends. It is a key to being successful. Chefs naturally want to accommodate people, but they must also learn to set aside time for themselves. I have been inspired by Spencer Johnson's book *Who Moved My Cheese?* It provides a wonderful little allegory about how to confront and adapt to change in the workplace. It got me to think about change in a positive light rather than as something to dread, and encouraged me to think in the long term rather than in the short term.

Sleep is Repair Time

There are 24 hours in a day, and I sleep 8 of those hours. I have 16 waking hours remaining and I don't want to work 14 of these. When I work 8 hours I am much more productive and I have 6 hours to myself to do as I wish. Although it was not easy to allow myself personal time, I came to realize that it was absolutely necessary. People often ask me how I get so much done? The answer is easy. If I'm well rested, and I have time for myself, I can come to work in the morning and be far more productive and efficient as a result.

Communication Causes Success

Communication via technology also contributes to the secret of my success. I have developed a time saving practice that assists me in problem solving. Using constant e-mail communication, I am able to keep the door open for dialogue and to at times solve problems before they happen. People often feel more comfortable informing me of potential issues using e-mail. Questions and concerns may relate to how a class might get new aprons or how the next group will subsequently use them. Whatever the issue, e-mail helps to simplify the path to communication and to keep me ahead of the problem. The reward for this exercise is extraordinary. I can address rumors or issues before they get too big and actually do any damage.

My Leadership Style Comes From Who I Am

I've developed a proactive leadership style because I don't like conflict. I cannot imagine throwing a pan at someone to manage their behavior. My philosophy at Cullinard is to nurture rather than to intimidate. I work best that way, and I believe that I can get the best from people with whom I work in this same manner. If I stand screaming at someone to cook a product such as a steak, medium rare, and they panic, the outcome can only be a steak that is overdone. We have enough exterior stress in our lives without creating our own. I try to build loyalty, trust, and an environment in which people feel safe. For me education is helping others. I teach people to "see it, own it, and fix it." Very simply stated, this means shifting responsibility to self.

I believe that it is difficult for new faculty members to assume the role of educator because they do not have a frame of reference upon which to base their behavior. At first they attempt to employ the same management techniques that they used in industry, but they soon learn that these methods are not effective in the academic arena. The bottom line is that we are about education, and learning is not always limited to student learning. Both students and faculty come to us with the belief that this is the best choice for them at the moment. With this in mind, we must remember that commitment and respect on the part of both are integral to success.

CASE DISCUSSION

Chef Bosich uses a systems approach in her classroom. She is committed to creating a positive environment for those in her charge. The management paradigm that she employs encourages people to want to do their best. The following questions will help to analyze her management philosophy.

CASE QUESTIONS

1. Does Chef Jill have a basic system of consequences for infractions that may occur?

2. Outline and discuss her leadership philosophy. Can you list at least three elements that contribute to her style?

3. What are the methods she uses to motivate others?

4. Which elements would motivate you as a student?

5. Are there any down sides to her strategies?

Jill Bosich is Dean of the Culinary Institute at Cullinard of Virginia College, Birmingham, Alabama

---

The real and hard work of the teacher is too often hidden from public view.

Rosetta Cohen, **A Lifetime of Teaching**

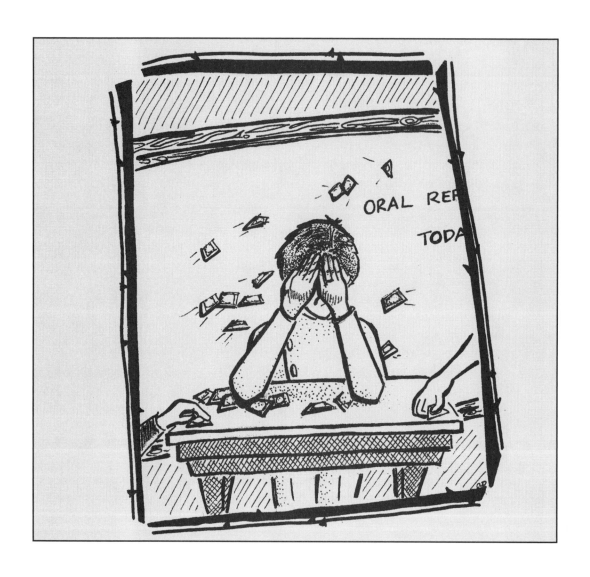

I Thought That Teaching Was Going To Be Easier

Getting Ready for Students

So here I am. I found my way to the kitchen classroom. What am I doing here? I was prepared to be a chef not a teacher. I have no preparation in teaching. I hope my ominous feelings aren't predictors of the amount of success or failure that I will experience here. How difficult can it be to teach? My responsibility is to teach all of the food classes, all of the *garde-manger* sections, and the basic and advanced food preparation sections. Even though I'm working on two campuses, I have only 20 students. How bad can it be? In fact, now that I think of it, it looks pretty easy. As a student, I perceived teaching as giving out assignments and presenting lectures. I can do that. I just attended a classroom management seminar with a great teacher, and so I feel armed and ready to go.

The Descent Into Teaching Hell

Was I ever in for the surprise of my life! Everything is working against me. I am too young to be in this job— and while it's not fair, that's working against me. I have never experienced this lack of respect before. Students act in ways that I find blatantly disrespectful. They don't bother to open their books in class when we are going through the text; nor do they bring pen and paper. They are late, they are absent, and they show a complete lack of respect for me. Anything that is considered unprofessional behavior is part of their repertoire. They talk out of turn, roll their eyes, accuse me of not knowing anything, misbehave in lab, and they come in looking like complete slobs, even though I have param-

9

eters on the syllabus for these behaviors. I'll bet they have never even read the syllabus. Why did I even bother preparing one?

Recently, I had one of the most horrible days in my beginning teacher career. My students had a project that they were supposed to have worked on the entire semester. Not only were all the projects poor, they were absolutely horrible. A majority of the class was one half hour to forty-five minutes late. Several students came in wearing the same clothes they had been wearing two days prior, and smelling like the Jack Daniel's Distillery and the Marlboro Factory all rolled into one. They were covered in dirt, alcohol spills, and God only knows what else. One young woman had to leave to go to the hospital due to premature labor, and the rest were lying on the tables moaning. The groups were disorganized and not ready to present their work. I had my first outburst of the semester. I was so angry and felt that I had been taken advantage of. I was almost in tears.

After my tirade about their lack of respect, the groups preceded to make their presentations. One of the groups that I thought had some promise, turned out to be an unbelievably catastrophe. Their presentation simulated a talk show on which some famous chefs were visiting and talking about themselves and their food. The host of the show, one of my brighter students, suddenly screamed something about a commercial break, at which point he yelled out: "Merry Christmas, and have safe sex!" Then hundreds of condoms came flying into the audience. I was sitting in the middle of a circle of Gold Coins and Trojans. Some of the students were crawling around on the floor collecting them exclaiming: "You can never have too many!" It was at this point that I realized that this isn't a culinary school; it is more like a halfway house for those who have been raised by wild animals. I was stunned. It is usually difficult to shock me, but at this juncture I was speechless. I just sat there surrounded by condoms wondering what if any of this had to do with food or learning. Maybe they aren't here to learn; at least I didn't think so that day. I realize that I have been becoming more and more of a babysitter and social worker (listening to all of their problems), and less of a teacher. Once again I am at a loss.

Trying to get Control

I have tried to get control of the class. The rules are getting stricter and stricter. Now I am at the point of wondering how much further I can go. I am not the top dog here. I don't get to say how far is far enough. It seems different than other programs. Where I went to school a person could actually be expelled. These kids can basically show up, sign their name on something, and somehow pass a course. It is this process that I find deeply disrespectful. If I were a man would they treat me this way? The other faculty in this program are men in their 40s. There is a small core faculty in this department. Students see us more than they typically see other faculty members. They call my teaching partners, Chef. They call me by my first name. I am short, blond, and I am not that much older than they are. I am 26 years old, going on 27. Why is it that I can say the same things that the men say and have students ignore me? Don't misunderstand me; they behave badly with the men too, but not quite to the extent that they do with me. In a recent evaluation, one of my students told me that he acted better for the men because he could not imagine me jumping over a table and smacking someone. Do they really think that the men will cause them physical harm, and therefore behave for them? Is it a different presence or gender that I need to get their respect?

Where Is the Support System?

Possibly the biggest surprise of my ill-informed impression of teaching has been the lack of support from administrators. I had assumed that they would be there for me. That's what it had looked like from the "outside world." This was a completely erroneous assumption on my part. Also problematic, in my opinion, is the lack of any semblance of uniformity among colleagues when it comes to classroom policies. All of our policies are different. Our being on the "same page" would resolve many of the problems. Because we all have our own policies, these 18 year-olds enjoy taking advantage of us by playing us one against the other as teenagers commonly do with their parents. If they don't get something from me, they go to the others. This has been their consistent pattern. If it were up to me I would send them home when they show up late. I have tried that, and although it works sometimes, the excuses run deep. I could write a book of excuses! "The bus didn't pick me up; my car wouldn't start; my alarm didn't go off!" Things happen every single day of their lives, and I don't know where to draw the line. I am at a point now where I guess I am tired, and I am trying to pick and choose my battles with them. I have three more months left with these kids, and I want to get it over with. They formed an opinion of me on day one and they haven't taken the time to see if it is at all accurate. That doesn't mean that I am not going to try to change their view. This generation seems different though. They don't look at life the same way that I viewed it when I was a student. If I did not show up for class or failed to take a test, there were consequences. They are so apathetic, yet at the same time they claim to know it all.

Things Are Only Getting Worse

Before Spring Break things had gotten really bad around here, so I thought I would try to do a mid-term evaluation on an individual basis. To go face-to-face with them was not an easy decision. I brought each of them into the office and told them they could say whatever they wished about me, about themselves, about their fellow classmates, or concerning the situation around here. I asked them to do this in a professional manner and to provide possible solutions to the problems. Prior to this, I had been doing written evaluations and trying to think of ways to remedy the situation. Finally, I came to the conclusion that it was really up to them. I had done as much as was humanly possible. The evaluations were very good. Every conversation that I had with students was excellent, and I was encouraged. However, I knew this was only the beginning. I am not naïve enough to believe that one conversation was going to make all the difference.

When we returned from Spring Break the situation became just as negative as it was prior to the interview/evaluations. Their behavior was sophomoric to say the least. Although I had had discussions with them and had spoken to them about proper classroom decorum, they continued to discuss topics that were not appropriate in this environment. I guess I am confused because during the evaluation meetings, they had all agreed to improve their behavior. I can't kick them all out, although I would like to at this point.

These are very difficult and trying times. Everything has gone down hill. I'm tired, and I feel that all is pointless. I

leave work every day feeling that I have accomplished nothing. While I don't put a lot of weight in many of the things
they say, I'm still hurt by their comments and their inap-
propriate decorum. There is nothing quite comparable to a
group of students telling a teacher that they think she knows
nothing and that she is not teaching them well. But it all
comes back to one thing, they are apathetic. The harder I try,
the worse it gets.

Having been in school many years and having seen so many
teachers in so many different situations, many beginners
think they know what it is like to teach. But, alas, it fools them.
The teacher's side of the desk is different. Behind it are hidden
demands and subtleties, which are quite unexpected.

Kevin Ryan, **Biting the Apple**

CASE DISCUSSION

To empathize with this beginning teacher who appears to have so little available to her in terms of coaching is natural. Although novices often experience some problems in the classroom, her situation appears to be one that is extremely frustrating. The fact is that learning to control a class and to motivate students at the same time is one of the most demanding tasks there is.

CASE QUESTIONS

1. Is this young teacher at fault, or is she a victim of the rogues that call themselves her students? Defend your answer.

2. Is the school to blame for this situation or is it society's lack of respect for the teaching profession that has created such a mindset? Explain.

3. What has this young teacher learned regarding the role of teacher? How can she communicate that her priority is teaching, rather than befriending students?

4. How can she maintain consistent discipline in her classroom? Are her boundaries clear?

5. What consequences can she set in place to decrease student infractions?

6. What are some of the ways in which this teacher can analyze these classroom issues and make sure that she is on solid ground in preparation for the next academic year?

7. What three classroom principles could this teacher use as a framework for building class rules?

8. How does a teacher set the tone for the learning environment?

9. How do teachers motivate while they teach?

10. How do teachers model professionalism?

11. How can teachers be themselves and honor their own style of teaching?

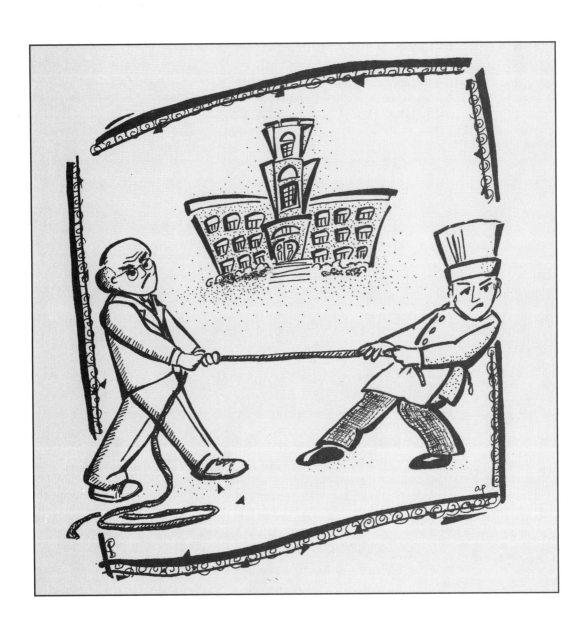

Leaving Industry for Teaching

Having come from the long hours demanded in industry, I thought teaching in a community college setting would be an easy adjustment. I was in search of a personal life and a family life that had been an impossible goal to achieve working in industry. I worked every holiday and every weekend, and these days stretched into the evening hours— 70 hours a week was the norm. My family life suffered. My wife became ill, and my children were growing up without a father. I loved working as a chef in a restaurant because I had the best appliances, a comfortable budget, and control that allowed me to achieve the high standards that I had set. I left all this in an attempt to bring balance to my life. As a chef educator I achieved balance, but I got many other surprises as well.

Industry has a built in respect for chefs. What they say goes, and people aspire to be the chef. There is respect for their expertise—they set the bar as to the goals that are to be achieved. In the community college environment however, people have very little idea of what it is that culinarians do. Sometimes we are thought of as "creative types" with the connotation of "weird." This perception was quite different from the way in which I had previously been viewed. I have been surprised to feel both misunderstood and devalued in my current role. It is true, that there is more job security here, and I do have time for family life, but I am paying a high price as well. I find it stressful and disappointing that those who are in authority have virtually no concept of what it is I am trying to accomplish here as well as what defines me as a chef.

Chefs are Perfectionists

To be a chef is to be a perfectionist. It can be said that the history of cooking is the history of excellence. Each plate prepared, as well as the overall appearance of the kitchen, reflect a chef's standards. Guaranteeing that each student completes the program with the highest aspirations of providing quality and service is my personal goal. But, the "lowering of the bar" to retain students continually threatens that goal. The message is not so subtle. We don't exist without students, and some of those who come to us have a poor idea of what it takes to be a chef. Some don't last a month. Cooking looks easy after one has mastered it. Watching others cook can provide an inaccurate picture of what is called for on the job. Chefs work notoriously long hours and are literally on their feet for 10 hours at a time, particularly at the beginning of their careers. The lifting involved also takes its toll, and many chefs have back problems. Cooking is a very physical endeavor.

Clash of Cultures

In addition to adjusting to the changes in status of a chef in industry to one of a chef educator, I have had the unpleasant experience of working for administrators who have little compassion for instructors who belong to unions. Since I have been in this community college system, I have never seen a president who did not have an anti-union mentality. Administrators, in general, are uncomfortable with the union and they try to keep their distance, which makes for an adversarial situation between instructors and administrators. Not only is there a basic misunderstanding of the expertise of culinarians, there is also a conflict between the standards of The American Culinary Federation and what administrators see as the implementation of those standards. When instructors are constantly told to lower their standards to retain students, programs die because the reputation of the institution goes down. Administrators are typically educators, and community college teachers are often individuals who have come from industry. When administrators speak "educational jargon", and instructors speak industry language, there is a lack of communication as well as a fundamental difference in values.

Community colleges don't model their management after business protocol, and that can be frustrating to the chef instructors who have come from industry. Because our administrators do not come from the business community, they do not understand the value of the credentials, the skills, or the degrees and certifications, that are respected in the outside work world. Nor do they grasp the value of the relationship with industry in building and maintaining quality programs.

No one seems to value good Teaching

In spite of all of the difficulties between management and instructors, the lack of respect for teaching is my biggest surprise. What is it about teaching that so few seem to value? Granted it may look simple, but it's not. Teaching looks easy because of the long hours that go into preparation time, which makes the delivery appear to be so facile. Preparing for one class session can take up to three hours. Making sure that the objectives are clear, the materials are ready, the lecture notes are thorough and easy to understand, and then teaching, and grading material afterwards is tremendously time consuming. I am in a situation where I am the only chef educator in my program (although this is a rather atypical community college model), and this makes for a demanding workday.

After all is said and done, I must admit that I value teaching and would not change my career. Administrative support would simplify my job and it would reassure me that they see some merit in what I do. The limited regard for the time, energy, and expertise needed to teach well is not acknowledged. Administrators rarely visit our program. In industry, "apprenticing" means watching an expert closely. It is just the opposite here. When we suggest methods to save money and ways in which administration might support us, we are not heard. Demands are made on us that they would never make if they were to walk a mile in our shoes. This whole academic management paradigm constantly reminds me that "I'm just a teacher, and that I am replaceable." I guess it would be accurate to say that historically teachers have been devalued and the complexity of their job greatly minimized.

Dealing With Disappointment

Since I see no immediate changes on the horizon, I must decide what to do. My choices are to go back to industry, to adjust to this management system, or to look for a teaching position somewhere else. Returning to industry is not a viable choice for me at this time because of my need to maintain a sound family life. Looking for another teaching position seems like giving up on something that I have worked so hard to achieve. My practical choice is to adapt to working with the present administration while maintaining a stance to guard the program's high standards.

Mechanized and often artificial divisions of labor promote closed relationships and heighten destructive conflict.

Donna Markham, **Spiritlinking Leadership**

CASE DISCUSSION

This chef is describing a community college system that appears to have a tremendous internal communication problem. The community college system plays a vital role in providing students chances that many might not otherwise have. In this sense, public education serves as a equalizer of opportunity. Because of the overwhelming demands placed on both administrators and instructors in these systems, it is easy to understand how both parties might be frustrated and find it easier to close their doors to input. What can chefs do to open the lines of communication?

CASE QUESTIONS

1. How can chef educators encourage the support of their administrators?

2. What is the definition of a "professional"?

3. What are some ways that chefs can influence the retention of students?

4. What information can be utilized to better inform potential culinary students of what it takes to be a chef?

5. What are ways that chefs can nurture their love of teaching and still prevent burnout?

6. What are some resources that chef instructors might use to create a less adversarial environment?

7. What are some communication devices that could be used to diffuse this tense scenario?

8. How can chefs decrease their feelings of isolation?

9. Do chefs have realistic expectations of their employers?

10. How can chefs begin to change the culture of their workplaces?

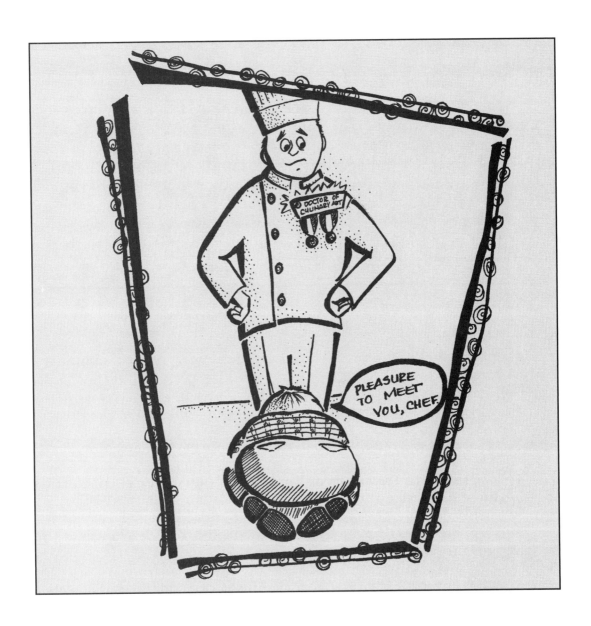

22

So You Want to be a Pastry Chef?

I grew up in the absolutely poorest of conditions that a person could ever dream of. I realized soon enough, after my years in high school, that I would have to figure out what to do with myself. There came a time when I had to say: "I need to make a decision about my future; I have got to make a living." I enlisted in the navy and was enrolled in chef's school. Soon after that I became a cook on board an oil tanker. When I left the Navy I felt that my artistic ability could be further developed if I were to train to be a pastry chef.

My apprenticeship began in 1958. Two years later, I saw an advertisement in a Swedish newspaper, placed by the man who owned Astra Pharmaceutical. He was interested in having someone come to the United States to set up a Swedish Pastry Shop. And so I asked my wife, "Would you like to go to the United States?" And she said, "Why, no." And so we did. We tried to think of this voyage as an adventure. In 1965 I met an individual by the name of Joe Amendola (from the Culinary Institute of America) at a culinary show in Boston, and he piqued my interest in becoming a vocational educator. I then decided to complete a degree in vocational education, which was required in the state of Massachusetts to teach vocational education. I was also required to become an American citizen.

Building a Certification Program for Pastry Chefs

Soon after this, I had the opportunity to help open a vocational arts department in Charlton, outside of Worcester MA, where I stayed for about three and a half years. One night at 11:00, I received a phone call from a superintendent who asked me to come to Cape Cod to serve as Director of Foodservice and Chairman of Culinary Arts. I wrote curriculum and surrounded myself with teachers whom I also felt were very good chefs. In 1978, I was hired by the Department of Education for the State of Massachusetts as an Education Specialist for Culinary Programs. The following year, I began my career at Johnson & Wales as Department Chairman of the Culinary Arts Bake Shops.

Four years later, I approached the president of Johnson and Wales University and asked him if he would be interested in supporting a program in pastry arts. The majority of pastry chefs in America at that time were European trained. Whenever I would be in a fine hotel or restaurant I consistently saw the European influence in the pastry they prepared. Little by little the idea of a pastry arts program began to attract interest. It did not happen overnight because we needed facilities to accommodate this program and the students as well. It was projected that we would have to have 60 students to make the program feasible, and we recruited only 13 at the time. Such low numbers were initially quite discouraging, but I refused to abandon my dream, and finally the program took shape.

We began with 4 instructors and within a year we had attracted 60 students to the two-year degree program. We now had more problems because we did not have the facilities in which to properly train these students. So during that summer we built a facility and hired more teachers. When I left the school in 1998, I had 26 pastry chefs and over 500 students in four different locations (Providence, RI, Norfolk, VA, Charleston, SC, and Miami, FL) People throughout the United States now look to the Johnson & Wales Pastry Arts Program as one of the best in the country.

Bringing the European Ideal to the States

Americans didn't know how to make pastry. They had limited vision. Their idea of pastry was white bread, hamburger rolls, and icing for cakes. It was very discouraging. In Europe at the time, people apprenticed for at least five years to learn the art. To study in America and to call oneself a pastry chef was unthinkable. Two years in a vocational school in America or a technical school was really just the beginning. An apprenticeship program would still be required in order for someone to be taken seriously as a pastry chef. Those who wished to be pastry chefs in Europe had to pass the apprenticeship examination, which entailed a mastery of skills designated by the trade institutions in Sweden, Germany, and Switzerland.

What Does it Mean to be a Pastry Chef?

The chef was always the person with the white hat. The earliest chefs came here from France and studied under Escoffier. French food at that time was the prime food in terms of cooking, ingredients, and taste. That has somewhat changed in the last 20 years. French food today is often considered to be too rich. So the French chefs have lost the "I am a French chef; I am from the Escoffier tradition" ego. In any country today including Germany, Switzerland, and Sweden, formal education is what is valued. Whether someone is a pastry chef or a master pastry chef really doesn't mean much anymore, although salaries still vary depending on the title.

Getting the Master Pastry Chef Certification

Prior to leaving Sweden, I had thought of pursuing my master chef certification, but I had not had the time to do so. Twenty years later, I wrote to the accrediting board telling them of my interest in acquiring my Master Pastry Chef Certification. So began a trail of correspondence that would prove my accomplishments. Eventually the Consul of the Swedish government informed me that the Ambassador of Sweden would meet me in Boston to award me my certificate. I made history. I was the first person to ever receive certification while not living in Sweden. The by-laws were changed, and now other chefs can also be certified if they qualify. Imagine this, it only took 38 years from the time I completed my apprenticeship certification until the day I received my master chef certification. Today, Johnson and Wales University does a tremendous job of preparing would-be chefs in two and four year programs depending on the certification desired. The old type of apprenticeship is on the way out, and relationships between students and teachers are healthier.

Servant Leadership and the Superego

The attitude of the chef towards others has changed tremendously since I began working years ago. The idea of the "chef's ego" came from Europe where the chef was considered king. But when I began teaching at Johnson & Wales my attitude changed completely, and I began to realize that cooking and life itself were not about ego. After many years of mastering the fundamentals, I began to think about how to motivate and educate students. I focused on what it was like being a poor kid in vocation education. At 16, I had not known what to do with myself, and although the times had changed, kids were still looking for their niche. So instead of being the "king of the kitchen," I began to serve them. I was there to help students understand that this was going to be their career connection.

When I hired instructors they would want me to look at their resumes. I would peruse them and then ask: " Do you have an ego?" Surprised at the question, they would hesitate before they responded. I would tell them that if they had an ego and they wanted to teach at this school, they had to leave it home every day. Forgetting one's ego does not mean a lack of pride or competitive spirit. I loved to compete on the culinary olympic teams, but I never thought of myself as a star. Instead, I was grateful for having been awarded such a great opportunity and felt a sense of pride in making an appearance with the other team members.

As a joke. I once had the titles Director, Manager, and Doctor of Culinary Arts Lars Johansson, monogrammed on a chef's jacket that I was to wear to a food show. Shortly after I arrived there, I was visiting with acquaintances when a young culinarian who read my jacket knelt down before me. My wife laughed when I told her the story and reminded her that all had gone as planned. This young man now teaches at Johnson & Wales.

Anticipatory socialization can be thought of as the mental act of "trying on" a role inside one's head and imagining what it might be like to actually hold the role oneself.

Dan Lortie, **Schoolteacher**

CASE DISCUSSION

Chef Johansson was a pioneer in bringing the European pastry ideal to the United States. In addition to this major accomplishment, he wrote curriculum and developed the pastry program at Johnson and Wales University that began with 13 students and has grown to number 500. The following questions can be used to help analyze the many stages that a chef goes through in developing a professional career.

CASE QUESTIONS

1. What attracted you to the food industry in the beginning?

2. How is being a chef educator different from what you thought initially?

3. What are the many roles that a person has to complete before actually becoming a chef?

4. Besides being a chef, what other roles can a person have in the foodservice industry?

5. What are the hidden difficulties of being a chef?

6. What are the actual responsibilities of an executive chef?

7. For what reasons do chefs leave the field for other work?

8. What does it take to build a culinary program?

9. What are three personality traits a chef must have to remain successful in the industry?

10. What are three personality traits necessary in becoming a successful chef educator?

Lars Johansson, Swedish Pastry Chef, is Director Emeritus of the International Baking and Pastry Institute at Johnson & Wales University

Part 1
Activities and Points to Ponder on Teaching Strategies, Teacher Burnout, and Classroom Management

Activity # 1: Book and Film Suggestions

The following books and films address relevant areas for learners. Their focus is on topics such as learning, psychological maladjustment, and behavior modification

In addition to this list you may select other resources that are approved by the instructor.

Books:
The English Teacher Who Couldn't Read by J. Corcoran
The Broken Cord by M. Dorris
Ain't No Makin It by J. MacLeod
How Children Fail by J. Holt
The Invisible Children by R. Rist
Among School Children by T. Kidder
I Know Why the Caged Bird Sings by M. Angelou
Makes Me Wanna' Holler by N. McCall
Murphy's Boy by T. Hayden
Cry Softly! The Story of Child Abuse by M. Hyde
Genie by R. Rymer
And Still We Rise by M. Corwin

Films:
To Sir With Love
Dangerous Minds
For The Love of Nancy

Type a one-page description of the circumstances that the principal character in the book/film experienced.

Topics of discussion may include—What made the character experience negative psychological development? What was wrong with this learning situation? How did the book/film helped to enrich your understanding of people and the way they might function in a school setting?

Activity # 2 Points to Ponder— How to Increase Attendance and Punctuality (other than by reducing grades)

1. Give quick and frequent quizzes as soon as class starts. If students are absent, they may make up quizzes on their own time.

2. Use in class writings as participation points. These are cued off the lesson so that students will find it difficult to make up this work if they miss class frequently. Yet, you may allow them to make up work so that you will be perceived as cooperative and fair. Students would rather find a way to come to class on time than to put in personal time later.

3. Make classes difficult enough. Students should not be able to pass without attending class regularly.

4. Keep attendance conscientiously. Take it at the beginning of every period.

5. Reward good attendance. At the end of each grading period offer percentage bonus points for those with limited absences.

6. Teach from the beginning of the period to the end.

7. Use class time wisely. Move it along, and use class time to teach what they can't teach themselves.

8. Stand at the door and greet them when they arrive or as they leave. Connection and caring promotes attendance.

9. If you want success with attendance and tardiness hold students accountable for missing class or arriving late.

10. Most importantly, model what you expect from them. Be on time and don't miss class.

Activity # 3 Points to Ponder—
Facts About the Brain

✔ The brain can deal with 5-7 pieces of information at a time (the average is five).

✔ The brain begins with information and then accepts or rejects it for further processing.

✔ For learners to retain something in long-term memory it must

MAKE SENSE + MAKE MEANING

✔ Meaning has the greater impact on retention.

✔ The brain can never make sense and make meaning at the same time.

✔ Build instruction first around the information, then around what it means.

From *How the Brain Learns* by D. Sousa.

Activity # 4: Most Influential Person Paper

In his book *Schoolteacher*, Dan Lortie theorizes that by the time we are college freshmen we have witnessed 33,000 hours of teaching. He believes that this sets up potential teachers to think that they know what the job is going to be like. He refers to this "miseducation" as "anticipatory socialization." "Anticipatory socialization can be thought of as the mental act of "trying on" a role inside of one's head and imagining what it might be like to actually hold the role oneself." (Lortie, 1975)

In a one to two page paper, typed, and double-spaced, write about your "socialization" to teaching. Complete the following statements to help you get started.

1. My early role models in teaching were . . .
    a) helpful
    b) destructive
    c) influential
    d) inspirational

2. Now that I am teaching, I find that it is more difficult than . . .

3. What I enjoy immensely about being a teacher is . . .

4. The parts I dislike most about teaching are . . .

I could make the following changes in my career as a chef educator to promote a healthy lifestyle for myself ...

Activity # 5: Instructional Theory Into Practice: Lesson Design

Objectives: SWBAT-(Student Will Be Able To)

Purpose/Meaning: What does this have to do with the course? What does this have to do with life? Why are these the objectives?

Anticipatory Set: This is the part of the lesson where the instructor sets the tone for the lesson. This exercise is designed to open the brain. Three things contribute to such an activity: novelty, significance, and relevance.

The Set has multiple purposes:
To make the objectives clear
To set the tone for learning
To pique students' curiosity
To show them the standard for their work

Input: This part of the lesson is typically referred to as the content piece. This is the body of the lesson, which can include readings from the text, lectures, films, discussions, or any other resources that support the chosen objectives.

Guided Practice: This section of the lesson involves giving students a chance to master or practice what has been taught. This is done during class time, and it gives the instructor the opportunity to check for understanding.

Closure: This is when the teacher asks the students: What did you learn?

Independent Practice: This is the educational expression for "homework." It refers to work done outside of class. Independent practice (or homework) can be a practical skills exercise or an enrichment activity such as reading a book.

Students can present a lesson to peers and the instructor can at that time verify their understanding of the lesson.

Adapted from *Instructional Theory Into Practice* by M. Hunter

Activity # 6: Learning Style Conflicts: What Shuts the Gates?

Type One Learners

Dislike:
- ✔ Competition
- ✔ Teachers and/or instruction that is not personalized
- ✔ Pressure in any form
- ✔ To be put on the spot to perform
- ✔ Isolated skills that are not tied into meaning
- ✔ Lack of quiet thinking time
- ✔ Risk taking
- ✔ Colorless Environments
- ✔ Lack of harmony: teacher-student or student-student
- ✔ Criticism—even when it's constructive

When they rebel they:
Tune out and withdraw

Under stress they need:
Positive reinforcement; time to become centered

Type Two Learners

Dislike:
- ✔ Lack of structure
- ✔ Unknown expectations
- ✔ Group projects
- ✔ To perform creatively on the spot
- ✔ Information out of sequence
- ✔ Lack of right or wrong answers

✔ Disorganization

✔ Lack of thinking time

When they rebel they:
Become very critical and withdraw

Under stress they need:
Clearly defined structure, quiet thinking time

Type Three Learners

Dislike:
✔ Lack of hands-on work

✔ Written assignments

✔ Sitting and Listening

✔ Reading directions

✔ Information that is not practical to them NOW

✔ Drill and Practice

✔ Being Patient

✔ Group work that is not task oriented

When they rebel they:
Become impatient, aggressive and refuse to listen

Under stress they need:
To become involved in an independent task that is active, relevant and enables them to experience positive results

Type Four Learners

Dislike:
✔ Imposed structure—being told what to do

✔ Standard routines

✔ Repetition and drill

✔ Teacher directed activities

✔ Working alone

✔ Not being allowed to talk

✔ One way to do things

✔ Non-creative tasks

✔ Teachers without a sense of fun and humor

When they rebel they:
Sabotage authority, talk back, act out

Under stress they need:
To talk it out, to be responded to with warmth and humor, to generate options

Activity:

1. Ask persons on the faculty or in the class to define themselves as a Type One, Type Two, Type Three, or a Type Four Learner based on the above listed criteria.

2. Since we teach or lead out of our Learning Style, we often resist other methods. What changes would you need to make to be effective in each of the learning styles?

3. Another idea: Group students based on their learning style. This is a fun way to help people recognize their favorite way of learning. Allow them to complete a group task in their particular learning-style group.

From *Learning Style Conflicts: What Shuts the Gates?* by Victoria Smith Associates.

Points to Ponder # 7: Discipline Diagnostic

Use the 10% rule as a diagnostic. When experiencing difficulty with a student, address that individual privately. If there are two students involved, also speak to them in private. If there are three or more students involved, address the entire group. The following questions will help to diagnose the problem.

How many? If there is less than 10 percent of the classroom population involved, address it as an individual issue. If more than 10 percent are involved address it as a group issue.

Which one? Are the same people causing the problems? If so, you can address the few. If not, there is a systems issue.

What kind? What are people doing? Analyzing these behaviors helps the teacher to discover the reason for such behavior.

When more than 10 percent of the class does not comply, give group consequences that will encourage the remaining percentage of the group to pressure their peers to comply.

From *Discipline Diagnostic*. By M. Long

Activity # 8: Average Retention Rate After 24 Hours

Lecture 5 %

Reading 10%

Audiovisual 20%

Demonstration 30%

Discussion Group 50 %

Practice by doing 75%

Teach Others/Immediate Use of Learning 90%

What implications does this model have for teaching others?

From *How the Brain Learns* by D. Sousa

Activity # 9: Career Stages

Classroom management issues, poor pay, and experiencing a lack of status can all cause teacher burnout. Betty Steffy's work provides an instrument to measure the career stages of teachers.

Career Stages of Classroom Teachers

1. Anticipatory Career Stage	idealistic, energetic, creative, growing
2. Expert/Master Stage	self actualized, master of classroom control, you are evolving, you demonstrate a with-it-ness
3. Withdrawal Career Stage	1) Initial Withdrawal = in limbo, loyal but feeling neglected 2) Persistent Withdrawal = teachers are critical of the system, teachers are critical of other successful teachers, deny personal responsibility for the need to change 3) Deep Withdrawal = when teachers are hurting students
4. Renewal Career Stage	teachers feel reactivated, growing again
5. Exit Career Stage	teachers experience a shift in commitment, they feel nostalgic, have a need for recognition, are often very judgmental about the organization's needs

From *Career Stages of Classroom Teachers* by B. Steffy

In 1989 Betty Steffy wrote *Career Stages of Classroom Teachers*, a helpful book on how people experience their careers. In her research on teacher burnout, she asserts that five career stages are possible in a teacher's life. **Write a one- page paper, typed and double-spaced, on the stage that you think you are currently in and why you believe this to be so.**

Activity # 10: Developing Teachers

Author Cynthia Barnes gives a comprehensive look at the developmental stages of teachers as learners. In a two-page paper, discuss her findings in light of teachers that you have known. Also, identify and elaborate on your own growth stage as a teacher.

Perceptions of:	WAVE 1 DISCOVER	WAVE 2 INVENT	WAVE 3 PRODUCE	WAVE 4 REFLECT
TEACHER	I know; they don't. Performer responsible for selecting and delivering content Control oriented Unaware of relationships among learning variables	I know; do they? Creating own meaning Examining relationship between content and process	What do I know? What do they? Creating/ adopting new methods Experimenting with relation-ships between process and learners Dissatisfied	I know! We know, but we don't know we know. Facilitating own and others learning Reflecting on experimentation Audience
LEARNER	Naïve Listener Empty vessel Passive Audience	Needs to study, work, think harder Seems disinterested	Challenging subject Frustrated Brings much to learning process	Performer Active Self-directed Integral part of learning process

Activity # 10: Continued

Perceptions of:	WAVE 1 DISCOVER	WAVE 2 INVENT	WAVE 3 PRODUCE	WAVE 4 REFLECT
PROCESS	Telling=teaching Cover the material Methods borrowed from own education Convergent Teacher-centered	Telling with flair=teaching Inventing own style Methods adapted to suit unique style	Learning=doing Results-oriented Methods borrowed from innovative practice More important than content	Learning= transforming Reflecting upon methods, materials Actualizing Divergent Learner-centered
CONTENT	Content-oriented Unexamined Mine-belongs to me The truth Static; finite	Personal style-oriented Examination beginning a truth Sometimes contradictory, inadequate	Critically examined Vehicle for learning process Dynamic questions integrated with methods, needs of learners	Critically reflected upon Pared to only that needed to effect learning Perpetually acted upon by learner Puzzle

From *Developing teachers: When the student is ready: The developmental "waves" of teachers as learner* by C. Barnes

Activity # 11—Points to Ponder Will students come to class prepared?

Try these strategies for better results.
Make daily quizzes from sample unit exams and allow students the following choices:

1. <u>To complete the daily quizzes on their own</u>. If a student reaches a 90 percent mastery level on the daily exams, he/she need not take the comprehensive unit test.

or

2. <u>To complete daily exams with a partner</u>. Those who select this option must also take the comprehensive exam.

Activity # 12: Selling School to Yourself

Necessity sometimes obliges us to specialize in areas in which we have little or no interest. To make this task more palatable we should analyze the positive effects that might be derived from the experience.

We might ask:

1. What does this particular specialty offer that no other specialty does?

2. How does it differ from other fields?

3. What is of importance to you now and will also be in the future?

4. What do people who study and become specialized in this field do?

5. Who are some of the famous people in this area of expertise?

6. What is most painful about pursuing study in this area?

7. How can you motivate yourself and persist to master the material at hand?

Activity:

In a 5 minute presentation to your peers, articulate the answers to the questions above. Convince them of the merit of the area of specialization that you have selected.

Activity # 13: Sanitation, Nutrition, and Supervision

Questions will address three areas:

✔ Sanitation (yellow cards)

✔ Nutrition (green cards)

✔ Supervision (blue cards)

1.   Prepare 10 questions on each of the three categories. Make the questions as difficult as they might be on the certification exam.

2.   Write or print them legibly on small index cards.

3.   Write you name, the question, and the answer on the front of the card.

4.   Bring the completed index cards to class. Eg.

Chef Kelley

The four food groups include?

grains
dairy
meats
fruits and vegetables

Activity # 14 Self-Grading

1.   Write the letter grade you think you earned.

2.   Write the approximate number of hours that you spent on this project.

3.   Rate this assignment on a scale of 1-10 for its usefulness. (Ten being the most valuable.)

Have students grade their own food product immediately after it is prepared. As the chef you can then give your comments. This technique allows for feedback on how students see their work and how they perceive your standards.

Part 1
Books for Further Reading on Teaching Strategies, Teacher Burnout, and Classroom Management

References

Bliss, T., J. Mazur and J. Buzzard. *Elementary and Middle School Teachers in The Midst of Reform: Common Thread Cases*. Ohio: Merrill Publishers, 2000.

Cangelosi, J. *Classroom Management Strategies*. New York: John Wiley & Sons, Inc., 2000.

Charles, C. *Building Classroom Discipline*. New York: Longman Publishers, 1999.

Childs, J. *The Philosophy of John Dewey*. (3rd ed.) Illinois: Open Court Publishing Company, 1939.

Cohen, R. *A Lifetime of Teaching*. New York: Teachers College Press, Columbia University, 1991.

Creswell, J. *Qualitative Inquiry and Research Design: Choosing among the five traditions*. California: Sage Publications, 1998.

Dewey, J. and J. Boydston, J. eds. *The School and Society*. Illinois: Southern Illinois University 1976.

Dewey, J. *Experience and Education*. New York: Kappa Delta Pi, 1938.

Doyle, W. *Classroom Management: Making managerial decisions in classrooms*. Chicago: University of Chicago Press, 1979.

Dworkin, A. and M Lecompte. (1991) *Giving Up On School: Student dropouts and teacher burnouts*. Newbury Park: Corwin Press, Inc., 1991.

Eckert, P. *Jocks and Burnouts*. New York: Teachers College Press, 1989.

Freire, P. *Pedagogy Of The Oppressed*. New York: The Continuum Publishing Company, 1970.

Gehrke, N. *On Being A Teacher*. West Lafayette: Kappa Delta Pi Publications, 1987.

Glasser, W. *The Quality School: Managing Students Without Coercion*. New York: Harper Collins Publishers, 1998.

Gouinlock, J. ed. (1976). *The Moral Writings of John Dewey*. New York: Macmillan, 1976.

Greene, M. *John Dewey: Master Educator*. New York: Atherton Press, 1966.

Hunter, M. *Enhancing Teaching*. New York: MacMillan College Division, 1994.

Hunter, M. *Mastery Teaching*. California: Corwin Press, 1995.

Hunter, M. *Improved Instruction*. California: Corwin Press, 1996.

Kilpatrick, W. Dewey's Influence on Education. In P. Schlipp and L. Hahn eds. *The Philosophy of John Dewey* . Illinois: Open Court Publishers, 1939.

Kowalski, T., R. Weaver, and K. Henson. *Case Studies on Teaching*: New York: Longman, 1990.

Lacey, C. *The Socialization of Teachers*. London: Methuen and Company Press, 1977.

Lortie, D. *Schoolteacher: A sociological study*. Chicago: The University of Chicago Press, 1975.

Moustakas, C. *Phenomenological Research Methods*. California: Sage Publications, 1994.

Nouwen, H. *The Inner Voice of Love*. New York: Bantam-Doubleday Publishers, 1996.

Oakes, J., and M. Lipton. *Teaching to Change the World*. Boston: McGraw-Hill, 1999.

Palmer, P. *Let Your Life Speak*. California: Jossey-Bass Publishers, 2000.

Palmer, P. *The Courage to Teach*. California: Jossey-Bass Publishers, 1998.

Palmer, P. *To Know As We Are Known*. New York: Harper Collins Publishers, 1983.

Pitton, D. (1998). *Stories of Student Teaching: A case approach to the student teaching experience.* New Jersey: Prentice-Hall, Inc., 1998.

Ryan, K. et al. *Biting the Apple.* New York: Longman, Inc., 1980.

Sarason, S. *The Predictable Failure of Educational Reform.* San Francisco: Jossey-Bass Publishers, 1991.

Sizer, T. *Horace's Compromise: The dilemma of the American high school:* Boston: Houghton Mifflin Company, 1984.

Sousa, D. *How the Brain Learns.* California: Corwin Press, Inc., 2001.

Stake, R. The Art of Case Study Research. California: Sage Publications, 1995.

Steffy, B. (1989). *The Career Stages of Classroom Teachers.* Lancaster, PA: 1989.

Waller, W. *The Sociology of Teaching.* New York: John Wiley & Sons, Inc., 1932

Walsh, K. *Discipline for Character Development.* Alabama: R.E.P. Books, 1991.

Yee, S. *Careers in the Classroom: When teaching is more than a job.* New York: Teachers College Press, Columbia University, 1990.

.

Journal Articles and Studies for Further Reading on Teaching Strategies, Teacher Burnout, and Classroom Management

Barnes, C. *Developing Teachers: When the student is ready: The developmental "waves" of teachers as learner.* Paper presented at the International Faculty Development Conference, Vail, Colorado, 1992.

Billingsley, B. "Teacher retention and attrition in special and general education: A critical review of the literature." *The Journal of Special Education.* 27 (2), 137-174, 1993.

Chapman, D. "A model of the influences on teacher retention." *Journal of Teacher Education*, XXXIV (5), 43-49, 1983.

Gibbons, L, and L. Jones. " Novice teachers' reflectivity upon their classroom management. " Research/Technical Report, 1994.

Gold, Y., R. Roth and C. Wright. "The factorial validity of teacher burnout measures. *Educational and Psychological Measurement* 52, 761-769, 1992.

Hargreaves, A., and N. Jacka. "Induction or seduction? Postmodern patterns of preparing to teach." *Peabody Journal of Education,* 70 (3), 53-65, 1995.

Harris, S. " A mentoring program for new teachers: Ensuring success." NASSP Bulletin, 79, 98-103, 1995.

Hewitt, P. *Effects of non-instructional variables on attrition rates of beginning teachers: A literature review.* Paper presented at the annual meeting of Mid-South Educational Research Association. New Orleans: Livingston University Press, 1993.

Hlebowitsh, P. "The forgotten hidden curriculum." *Journal of Curriculum and Supervision.* 9 (4) 339-349, 1993.

Jesus, S., and M. Paixao,. *The "reality shock" of beginning teachers.* Paper presented at the International Conference of FEDORA, Coimbra, Portugal, 1996.

Long, M. *Discipline diagnostic*. Washington: Whitworth College.

Natale, J. "Why teachers leave." *The Executive Educator*, 18, 14-18, 1993. National Commission of Teaching and America's Future. "What Matters Most" teaching *for America's Future*. New York: Columbia Teachers College Press, 1996.

Sclan, E. (1993). *The impact of perceived workplace conditions on beginning teachers' work commitment, career choice commitment, and planned retention*. Paper presented at the annual meeting of the American Educational Research Association, Atlanta, GA, 1993.

Teacher Supply, Demand, and Quality Research Project. (1995). *Report Number 6*. Austin, TX: Education Agency, Division of Policy Planning and Evaluation, 1995.

Tusin, L. *Success in the first year of teaching: Effects of a clinical experience program*. Paper presented at the annual meeting of the Association of Teacher Educators, Michigan, 1995.

Victoria Smith Associates. *Learning Style Conflicts: What Shuts the Gates?*

Vonk, J. *Conceptualizing novice teachers' professional development*. Paper presented at the annual meeting of the American Educational Research Association, San Francisco, California, 1995.

Vonk, J. *Mentoring beginning teachers: Development of a knowledge base for mentors*. Paper presented at the annual meeting of the American Educational Research Association, California, 1993.

Leadership, Management, and Organizational Theory

EXPERIENCES OF CHEFS IN INDUSTRY

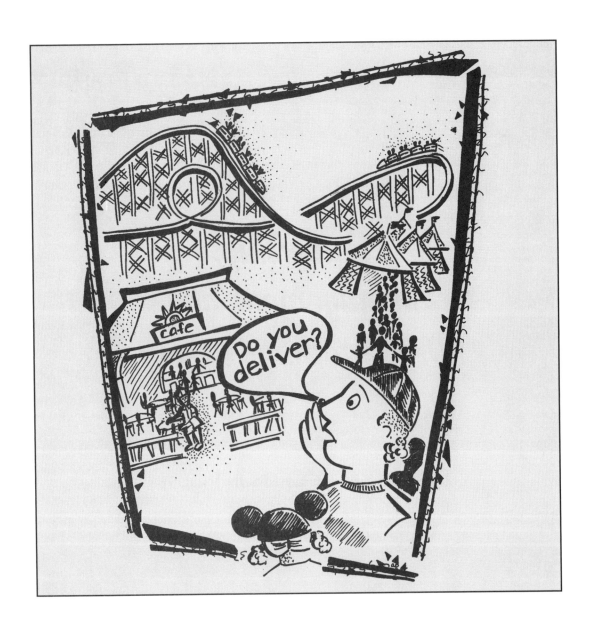

Being A Chef Manager at Disney Means Making Magic

Food is the Second Important Experience for the Guest

A chef who works for a corporation where food is not the primary focus must be creative enough to weave the food experience into the business' initial draw. Since I work in the entertainment industry, this is my primary challenge. My name is Shannon Johnson, and I am a Chef Manager at the Disneyland Resort.

When people think of Disney Theme Parks, they first think of attractions and entertainment, rather than of the restaurants housed on that property. Chefs who prepare food for corporations, in this case a theme park, have a different role than most other chefs, because people come to a theme park to have fun and to visit the attractions, and not necessarily to experience the food.

Working Around the Guest

There are several factors that must be considered in a theme park environment, and a chef must be aware of these to effectively prepare for guests. In a theme park the guests have come to play. They expect to have a wonderful experience and to be thoroughly entertained during their stay. Food is not their primary concern. In fact, guests often times forget to eat. We must create exceptional food experiences, and be ready at almost any time to provide guests with great food. For us, the question to answer is "how can we make sure that guests have the best experience possible in the limited time they have allotted to enjoy the food experience?"

Theme parks are notorious for long lines. When people have forgotten to eat, they have little desire to wait in a long line with their hungry children. To prepare for this, we use three types of targeted foodservice operations that are strategically placed throughout each park. The three types of locations are table service, buffeteria, and quick service. Within each of these categories there are numerous restaurant locations, each carrying the theme that is highlighted in that particular section of the park. These provide many choices to fit guests' needs. We know the hourly meal capacity for every restaurant, and the time necessary for each transaction. The facilities are designed based on a model of the number of people that they can serve per hour. From the transaction plan, we generate data that is plotted and forecasted, and which allows us to meet guests' demands. As a result, our guests are not inconvenienced by an incredibly long wait. In addition to capacity, we look at peak eating periods.

There are certain times during which guests eat at theme parks. Since they have a tendency to get wrapped up in their experience at the park, the traditional lunch period doesn't really exist. If a family gets to a Disney Park at around 9:00 or 10:00 am, and the kids are so excited about enjoying attractions, buying balloons, watching shows and having a great time, lunch may be delayed to 1:30 or 1:45 in the afternoon. For us, this impacts the traditional lunch period. In terms of planning, we must consider the irregular times of day that guests come to eat and we must be prepared to provide a consistently great experience, in an expedient manner, and at any possible moment. If we are unable to accomplish this, guests may forego eating, which means we have lost the opportunity to capture that meal and create a food experience.

Working at Disneyland is About Flexibility

Everything in a theme park is dependent upon the dynamics of the number of guests who visit on any given day. Most food locations are open for lunch and dinner; however, we are always ready to " flex" that operation. The hours we're open are based on the number of guests in the park. Certain periods during the year are slower than other seasons, so we are constantly adjusting to meet these demands. Consequently, our business is quite fluid. We carefully follow attendance trends and study guests' dynamics. At times this means that even the park's opening and closing hours vary. Disneyland is commonly open from 9:00 am until midnight; however, if it rains, the park may close much earlier. In the case of high winds, a restaurant location may become vulnerable to weather conditions and experience a fluctuation in attendance and operating hours.

Restaurant operators and chefs must be flexible in accommodating these changes. We purchase food products based on the forecasted attendance (the number of guests anticipated). It can be rather hectic when a large quantity of food has been purchased and the restaurant has to close because it starts raining. A closing can impact waste and spoilage, and as a result, greatly affect food costs. But we do try to maintain consistent location operating hours each day not to confuse guests.

In my first position at Disneyland, I was responsible for overseeing all food production for the New Orleans Square area of Disneyland. There were five restaurants within that one area and collectively they generated millions of dollars. My primary responsibility was to maintain a commissary kitchen underneath those restaurants. The facility was the ultimate food production basement. Our job was to produce a variety of 95 different fresh food products that went to the five restaurants. During that time it was important for me to learn how the park flexed in its hours of operations, not only from a food purchasing and production perspective, but also from a scheduling and human resource side. Working in that position prepared me for the flexibility that we in food service must have in order to cater to the needs of our guests.

The Life of a Chef Manager at Disneyland

Feeding large groups of people at Disneyland often demands a cast of 110 or 115 members in the kitchen during summer peak hours. For a chef, the hours are not as constant as they might be in a traditional setting—there tend to be peaks of long hours instead. During the holiday season and summer time, there are many special events that take place and turn a regular day into a very long day. Even though I get two days off a week, I consistently feel pressure to perform to the high Disney standards, and more importantly, to the expectations of our guests.

Working in a Union Environment as a Chef Manager

Currently, we have approximately 20,000 Cast Members (the term used for anyone who is employed), and about 5,000 of these people are in the food service business at the Disneyland Resort. All employees are members of a labor union. I was hired as a restaurant manager, and with my culinary background, my main focus was to improve food quality and food efficiency within the park environment. This is my first union experience and I find that it is an unusual environment for a chef to work in, since there is often no union involvement in the restaurant business. Sometimes management and the union are at opposite ends of the spectrum and the goal is to meet in the middle and to recognize that each side has a legitimate perspective. As a manager of a union business, I try to forget that there is a union and I take care of my Cast Members as if they were part of my "restaurant family".

Earlier in my career, I worked for a gentleman named George Kappler, who from a values perspective, greatly influenced my management style. His philosophy was to take care of people in a completely fair and even keeled approach. When I worked for him, he taught me how to treat others by going the extra mile and caring about issues that concerned them. In many ways, his philosophy relates to a model that we use within the Disneyland Resort. The guests, the employees, and the financial concerns make up a triangle. Keeping the triangle in balance creates a great organization. The Cast makes up the employee side of the triangle. If the Cast Members are unhappy or are distracted in other ways, this affects the financial side, and ultimately impacts the guests. Every decision is made with the triangle model in mind. If people are late for work, or restaurants run out of ingredients, the triangle is toppled.

Making a Profit as an Artist

Every chef is an artist trying to make a profit. As a chef, that is one of the magic parts of our job. The idea is simple—take the ingredients and make them into something special. Try to give the most mundane product a quality that it wouldn't otherwise have. As a chef, I might say "I am going to take this green bell pepper and make it the best anyone could imagine." There isn't as much magic in paying too much for the very best products and turning them into something so special that they're priced out of the market.

It has more to do with taking good quality products, and turning them into incredibly tasty foods. Sometimes chefs spend money on ingredients only to find that people don't identify with them, and so they may not sell. The magic artistry is made very clear to guests when common ingredients that they have in their own homes are presented in ways that they could have never imagined. The key to capturing a vast segment of the restaurant market is to impress with simple fresh ingredients and skill rather than with exotic ingredient snobbery. Once a large segment of the market has been captured with creative positioning of an otherwise basic product, then profit is just around the corner. Have you ever heard of a coffee shop called Starbucks?

Technology Makes for Interesting Food Possibilities

Eating in a restaurant is one of the few experiences that people have in which they don't sample the product before they purchase it. Guests are limited to reading a description on the menu and on the communication skills of the server. This puts a high value on the individual who describes the food. Food is more complex today than it was 50 years ago. The method of preparation, the diversity of the ingredients, and a descriptive copy must all be given on the menu. Writing about the food on a menu was once a simple task. Now there is an art in accurately describing to patrons what they are ordering. I try to anchor a menu on food that people know. This helps to limit possible confusion, and to make the ordering process and the dining experience a little more pleasurable. When people actually receive what they thought they were going to get; they can relate to it when they taste it. This is a big part of the enjoyment for a guest. There is nothing worse than ordering something and then thinking, " This isn't at all what I thought it was going to be." When an entrée costs $20.00, it can be even more disappointing. Employees understand the risks guests take when they order, and they attempt to make the dining experience one that is pleasurable. We try to keep the guests' thinking in mind. We make an effort to anticipate obstacles to a memorable dining experience, and once the obstacles are identified, we work in teams to eliminate them. These teams may include managers, chefs, Cast Members, and last but certainly not least, the guests.

We have a job to do, and it is about guest enjoyment. Selecting the best possible choice to accommodate guests is our mission. When I have issues such as kitchen Cast Members who are consistently late or absent, I must address these work habits. Everything that we do or don't do has an affect on the guest's experience. Everyone in the restaurant must understand this before a balance of great food and great service can be delivered.

"Stay on message" was drilled into my head by Mike Berry, former Disney Vice-president and current President of Barnes and Noble. One of the ways a chef can do this is by creating a standard that does not change so that an employee has a chance to "get it right." As chefs and managers, we need to give our employees the chance to "do right by" the guest with clear direction and clear standards of conduct. When there is too much change, people get confused and fear getting in trouble. Consistency also helps in producing a uniform product. Organizing the kitchen in a way that utilizes everyone's best efforts, is tremendously helpful for employees. Labor is becoming more expensive than food costs, so getting the best out of people plays a big role in the success of an organization.

Being a good manager means taking responsibility for communication. This is not easy because employees expect a lot from a leader. As my communication skills improve, my job becomes easier. A part of managing is helping people "to get on the same page" and to follow policies. This creates a better work force because workers know that infractions are taken seriously. This can also prevent more serious problems. A chef has to establish credibility, maintain consistency, and communicate effectively to be happy as a manager of people. I think that employees get excited if employers and supervisors are enthusiastic. The boss creates the culture of a work place, which must be more than a site at which to collect a paycheck. Having clear expectations of employees, following up, and holding everyone accountable is critical.

Being a successful chef has as much to do with business as it does with the artistry of food. Because chefs are artists, they are often inclined to get emotionally involved and passionate in everything they do. Passion is essential for a chef, but so is paying attention to the business. The business side is literally the admission ticket for a creative, successful chef. Cash flow must remain positive. Although the financial side is certainly taught in culinary school, the numbers may not always be realistic. Impromptu situations that occur in restaurants are not commonly covered in class. For example, when the market for fresh product goes up and down, and prices of goods go up, a chef cannot always raise menu prices to cover the loss and this could kill a business.

Envisioning the financial structure of a restaurant holistically is the key to managing fiscal performance. Chefs and managers, all too often, target one line or another on a profit and loss statement or another fiscal report, and forget to look at the big picture. All costs in a business are interrelated. The manager must find the combination of controllable costs that give a business the best opportunity for success. A fixed formula for managing a restaurant's controllable cost does not fit every situation. When one or more cost factors are volatile, it puts pressure on all the other costs. For example, if labor costs continue to spiral upward due to low unemployment or other factors, it is not wise to maintain the same food cost that was previously in place. Flexing the other controllable costs may help to weather the storm.

Spiritlinking leaders work to develop modified consensual strategies that leave the door open for the unexpected.
Donna Markham, **Spiritlinking Leadership**

CASE DISCUSSION

Chef Johnson has given us a look at what lies underneath the magic at Disneyland. He presents us with a comprehensive view of what it takes to prepare meals for thousands of guests. These questions will help to extrapolate his strategies.

CASE QUESTIONS

1. What types of unexpected financial scenarios might occur?

2. How can chefs be better prepared to run the business side of an operation?

3. How can chefs avoid thinking they won't be hurt by financial decisions?

4. What are 10 ways in which chefs can think of "the guest first?"

5. What are 20 skills that chefs need to be able to do to perform daily?

6. What are some communication strategies that chefs use to communicate effectively with others?

Shannon Johnson is a Chef Manager at The Disneyland Resort in Anaheim, California

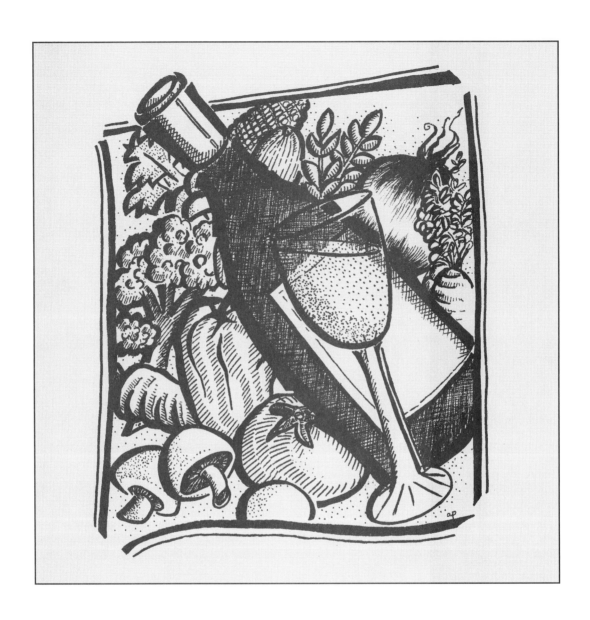

Vegetables as a Mainstay

Chefs Cook the Way They Eat

When I was young, I thought that I was invincible. I believed that I could live any way that I wanted and that I could eat whatever I pleased. When I turned 40 years old, I began to see things differently. I started to think about health as a lifestyle. Now I consume primarily vegetables, and a dramatically reduced amount of protein from meats. This new way of eating has encouraged me to experiment with vegetables in my cuisine.

The way chefs feel about food dictates how they cook and how they design their menus. My style is a bit more involved because I use vegetables as a mainstay and not just as a side dish. I offer a number of vegetarian dishes, pastas, rice and grains. There is such an abundance of products for chefs to choose from so it is easy to have a larder full of these ingredients. It is natural to create new dishes and to choose from a wide variety of ingredients because every chef wants to have something that others don't have.

Building Dishes and Menus

I begin the building of each meal on a particular wine. Every menu is built around the flavors and moods that present themselves in that wine. I have a very strong technical background. The school where I learned to cook trained students extensively in the basics, both in school and off site. To emphasize the importance of a well-rounded background, I use an analogy of the architect and the carpenter. An architect doesn't have to be a carpenter, but it sure helps if he or she knows carpentry because it makes it a lot easier for design elements to occur. I feel the same way about cooking; having a technical background gives me a stronger sense of what I can do in the kitchen.

I know where I am going with a dish without creating the dish in a laboratory setting. I sense the flavors in my mind before they exist. At the annual Boston Wine and Food Festival, we have 55 events, and in 12 years I have not prepared the same dish twice. The day before the event, I create dishes based on the flavor of the wines that are being shown. For example, if I am tasting a heavy oak Canard Chardonnay from California, I may pick up the elements of char wood, possibly pears, and a nice acidic balance of butter. With these as my basics, I come up with a dish that can work in one of three ways, it will be either be compatible to, or contrast with one of the flavors, or it may combine with all three flavors of the wine. I use these three elements to pair the wine and food. We then create the dish the actual day of the event. Food, of course, is best appreciated when experienced in the setting for which it was designed.

Crafting the Dish for the Customer

I also know my clientele and have a sense of their style, and this too influences my dishes. A very conservative guest will better appreciate a traditional offering, while a Randal Graham would much prefer a more creative approach to a dish. But in both cases, the wine and the food must work together.

Vegetables for Color, Health, and Variety

I cook with a variety of vegetables that are plentiful in the market place. Although nothing is cheap, vegetable costs are considerably lower than beef and fish. Even in Boston where fish is as fresh as it can be and usually plentiful as well, prices are high. I pay a premium price for vegetables because I use 80% organic product. I also order baby beet tops and a variety of other unusual vegetables that are a bit pricier. Obviously, my produce costs are higher than those of most chefs. I often spend as much, if not more, on vegetables than I do on meats and fish. A dish of codfish for example, might be accompanied by a variety of four vegetables. Whether I use wild asparagus, or beautiful black or white Rainier cherries, or other seasonal fruits they all contribute considerably to the depth and the texture of the plate. Chefs are increasingly incorporating external influences into the texture, composition, flavor, and presentation of their dishes.

People are Interested in Taste

When I began cooking at the hotel, I was able to offer one dish on the menu that had a vegetarian emphasis. After 12 years on site, 20% of the menu consists of vegetarian offerings. These meals are popular and they sell well, particularly at lunchtime when people like to eat lighter. Although many Americans today are better informed about healthy diets, they must still be encouraged to actually "eat healthy." In addition to looking attractive, meals have to be tasty to sell.

To enhance the flavor of vegetable dishes, I use fresh herbs and spices and employ cooking techniques such as charring, roasting, smoking, or flash searing. My goal is to prepare vegetable dishes in a manner that actually allows guests to forget that they are consuming more vegetables. The hotel's downstairs café alone, "does 200 covers" at lunchtime, and of these, 30 or more sales are from vegetarian choices. One of the most popular dishes we offer is a crisp fresh tortilla with very thinly sliced tomato, roasted spinach, and avocados, served with or without cheese. The tortilla is pinwheeled, griddled, and served with an accompaniment of wood-fired Hungarian spelt tabouli. We pride ourselves on knowing that our patrons are selecting vegetable entrées for their great flavor.

Business is Great!

Repeat business greatly contributes to our overall profit. Local clientele provide 87% of our income while hotel guests account for only 13%. An average of 1300 meals are served daily at an operation consisting of 7 banquet rooms and 3 restaurants. The average number of meals served daily has risen from 350 to 1300 per day in a twelve year period and sales have gone from $4,000,000 to $22,000,000 during that same time frame. The kitchen is staffed by 44 people.

"Dance With Who Brung 'Ya"

I like to cook and I get to do so fairly frequently. It is important to me to run an operation from the trenches. I have an organized kitchen in which I work side by side with my staff. Work keeps me energized and makes me forget the long hours that I invest in my job. Although many chefs eventually make the transition from chef to business administrator, I like to balance both roles. Being happy and having fun at work is as important to me as is making money.

Service, Flexibility, and Success

An important aspect in running a successful operation is flexibility in accommodating guests' wishes. At our restaurants, it is not a problem when customers wish to substitute accoutrements. Serving more or less of one food item or another, or a different combination of choices, is an easy request to satisfy. As chefs, we are here to provide our clientele with the best dining experience possible. Why not give guests what they like? Customer satisfaction is the foundation upon which a great reputation is built.

Being a good chef is being an alchemist, the seemingly magical craft of changing something into something better.

CASE DISCUSSION

Chef Bruce has shared with us the secrets of his success. Answering the following questions will help you to reflect on the numerous strategies and skills that he employs daily.

CASE QUESTIONS

1. What are some ways in which chefs can overcome their own bias for using more vegetables in dishes?

2. How can chefs get customers to try new foods?

3. How can chefs educate patrons about nutrition without turning them off?

4. In what ways have chefs successfully addressed changing the way their clientele eats?

5. What resources are available for chefs to learn about cooking healthier?

6. Plan three menus based on Chef Bruce's techniques.

Daniel Bruce is Executive Chef at the Boston Harbor Hotel

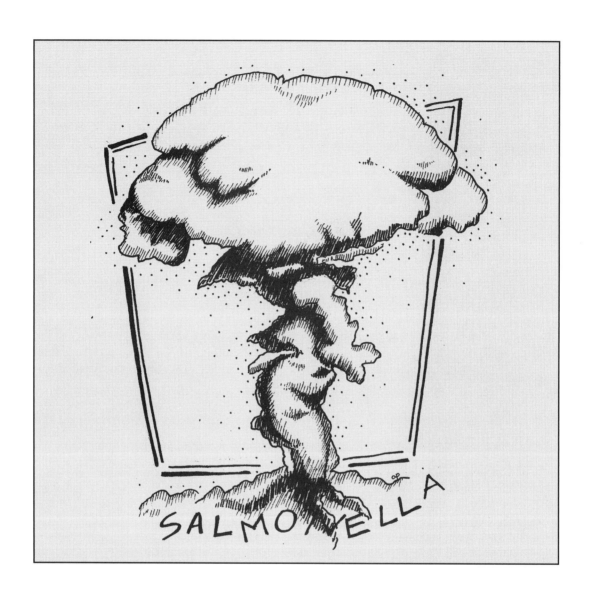

The Salmonella Scenario

I wasn't a Rookie

I was a graduate of The Culinary Institute of America, and I had apprenticed at the 1980 Winter Olympics held in Lake Placid, N.Y. I served as an Executive Chef in a well-known restaurant in Columbus, OH., and I also worked as a sous chef at a New England inn. Needles to say, I did not think that I might be the cause of a Salmonella outbreak.

A Five Star Job

In 1984, I was the Executive Chef at Hotel A. The Hotel was owned by an English company that had come to the United States to establish a quality hotel with European style. The property housed three restaurants and banquet facilities that could accommodate up to 10,000 people. The hotel was a 4 star, 4 diamond property. There were approximately 60 cooks and chefs who were scheduled to work throughout the day. On a busy day we often cooked 75 prime ribs. These were prepared in alto shams (a slow-cooking unit uniquely designed for this type of roasting).

A chef could set the temperature and time to slow cook the product and then reset the temperature and time to "hold" the product at a desired temperature. All meats were cut to specification, and all products were hand butchered, put into plastic bags, and sealed with twist tops. They were not shrink-wrapped. We worked with a state of the art meat company, we had handling procedures down to a science, and we used what I would classify as a tight system for cooking, roasting, and holding product. We never had a problem until the day that I decided to go on vacation.

Salmonella Poisoning

While I was away, the Director of Operations for the Hotel decided that he was going to offer an "All You Can Eat Lobster and Prime Rib Event". In order to do this, a lower quality of prime rib was ordered to keep food costs down. Because chefs are responsible for food costs and profits, the employees, in my absence, ordered a lower quality rib than our usual grade from a different wholesaler. They followed the same preparation procedures that had been in place and proceeded to serve the prime rib. At one site we served 450 people dinner, and of those, 60 people came down with Salmonella poisoning. Dinner patrons, managers, and guests in the hotel who had eaten the prime rib were infected. I returned from my vacation and walked into the middle of a nightmare. I was on my rounds when I received a call from the administration at the hotel who told me what had happened and requested that I report to the office immediately. After having spoken to the Director of Operations and with numerous chefs, I knew that the problem was indeed the roast beef.

A Media Fiasco Followed

I asked the local health inspector not to break the story to the media until we had all our facts together, and until we knew exactly what had occurred. From day one, I told him that the problem had to have originated with the roast beef as that was the only change that had been made in the kitchen. The numbers of people infected continued to grow. Eventually, I too got Salmonella. Most of our chefs (including myself) were removed from the facilities. We had to shut down The Café, where we had been generating $350,000-400,000 a week in sales. This was a considerable amount of money in the 1980s. I continued to work with the Health Department in an effort to identify the exact cause of the poisoning. Meanwhile, the local health inspector revealed the information to the news media and it was broadcast over all the television networks. As soon as the story broke, people stopped coming to the hotel and all the food related functions were being cancelled. The operational output of 10,000 meals per day dropped to zero. The media never let up. The health department, after having inspected a prime rib at the lab, shut down all foodservice operations. No food was to leave the hotel. Most of the chefs quit or moved to other positions.

**Our Errors
are Deadly**

Ultimately, it was determined that we had not cooked the roast beef properly. At the time, the Health Department was instructing foodservice establishments to cook roast beef at 140 degrees to 145 degrees F internal temperature for medium, and 150 degrees F internal temperature for medium well. We were instructed to slice the product and then reheat it. It was not advisable to serve the roast beef rare, but customers continually demanded to have their roast beef rare. So we decided to cook it at 120 degrees to 130 degrees F in an alto-sham (slow cooking oven unit), in an attempt to satisfy patrons.

Today we know that in order to kill Salmonella bacteria, strict temperature and time regulations must be adhered to. For example, rare roast beef is safe to serve at 130 degrees F, but it must be at that internal temperature for 121 minutes to kill the bacteria.

**The Real
Cause of the
Tragedy**

Some years later when I was watching 60 Minutes on television, they began speaking about a lawsuit that had been filed by all the hotels, nursing homes, and restaurants that had been shut down at the same time as our property due to the salmonella outbreak. The suits were against the same company that had sold us our contaminated beef. The Health Department had gone into their warehouse and had found salmonella all over, on meats and inside trucks. The meat was contaminated on the outside, and had we cooked it properly, we might have prevented the outbreak.

**I Couldn't
Buy a Job**

I couldn't buy a job. One day I was making over $60,000 as an executive chef, and the next day my career was gone. I was living a chef's worst nightmare. I went from a prestigious job in a prominent hotel to the unemployment line. I was devastated! I couldn't find a job as an executive chef because potential employers checked references. I worked construction for a while and eventually built up the funds and the courage to start my own catering business. I catered for prominent individuals and was eventually able to rebuild my reputation. The hotel continued to operate, but it never really sprung back from the stigma of a Salmonella outbreak.

The High Cost of Learning

It was clear that the Director of Operations had not followed my specifications and company procedures. I bought from a particular vendor and certain packinghouses because they were local companies who were known for their quality product. I could tour the plant any time I wanted to, and I knew that their quality control was excellent. I had local contacts and could guarantee the quality of my product to the customer. In addition to the careers that were destroyed, the hotel lost millions of dollars. Chefs sometimes do not realize that there is more to being a chef than just cooking.

The Bottom Line

The bottom line is temperatures and procedures are very important. Chefs must post and follow HACCP Flow Charts. Also, know your purveyors. Inspect the plants and be sure that appropriate quality control standards are in place. Keep accurate records of all inventory.

Restaurants and chefs sometimes assume that all businesses are conscientious. Many foodservice operations do not take appropriate precautions when receiving products to ensure food safety. Chefs get busy, they schedule improperly, and at times fail to train employees appropriately. When employees work 50 to 60 hours per week and lack training, catastrophes occur. Today we have laser thermometers to check the temperatures of frozen food products. This quick and efficient tool can be used to check a whole case of chicken in just a few minutes.

But in many restaurants today, there are hi-tech devices and improperly trained employees using them. The strongest lobbying power against stringent sanitation laws and certification requirements is the foodservice industry. Grocery stores and chain stores in particular are opposed to stricter laws because they would have to train employees and this would cost money. Sanitation concerns distinguish true professionals from those who are pseudo-professionals. National certification boards require 30 hours of sanitation training for chefs, because they realize that human life is valuable. All accredited programs and high school secondary accredited programs require such certification.

⊞❘❙

CASE DISCUSSION

This case study is included to demonstrate the necessity of quality control and the importance of education in the foodservice industry. The questions that follow address how chefs can guarantee product safety.

CASE QUESTIONS

1. What procedures are necessary in the foodservice industry to ensure product safety?

2. If beef is not usually a Salmonella culprit, how did such a catastrophe occur?

3. What precautions can chefs take to prevent outbreaks?

4. Which resources should chefs look to for temperature guidelines for cooking meats?

5. How can chefs guarantee food safety and maintain a controlled product cost?

For each of us lives in and through an immense movement of the hands of other people. The hands of other people grow the food we eat, weave the clothes we wear, and build the shelters we inhabit.

James Stockinger, as cited in **The Good Society**
by Bellah et al (1991, p. 104)

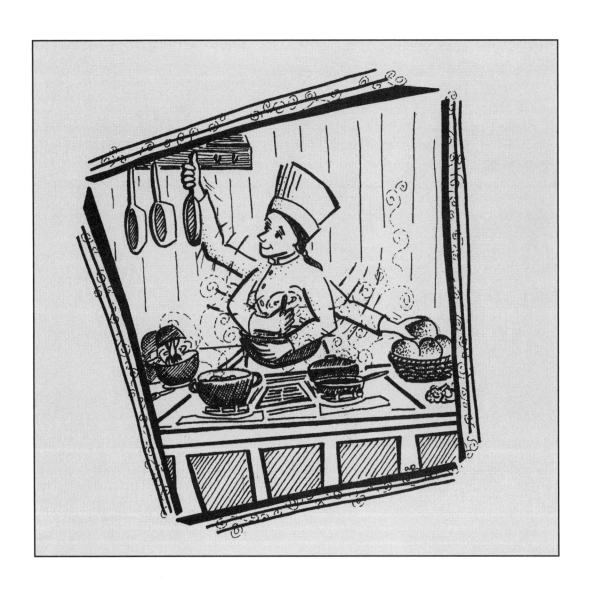

Why Aren't There
More Women Chefs?

Who are our Models?

When we contacted Sara Moulton, Executive Chef of *Gourmet Magazine*, founder of The New York Women's Culinary Alliance, and host of the Food Network's *"Cooking Live,"* and asked her why there aren't a greater number of women chefs, we struck up an interesting conversation on this topic.

What are the Numbers?

We asked Chef Moulton to estimate the number of women chefs in the workforce. She stated that she believes that there are fewer than 10% of chefs who are women if we use the general term chef, and an even smaller percentage if we speak about the "chef" as the individual who is actually running the kitchen.

The career does not appeal to women in part because of the limited number of female models in the industry. California, she believes, probably has the largest number of female chefs due to people such as Alice Waters, who have set the stage for other women. The West Coast offers great opportunities for women and men alike, and there are also a good number of female chefs to work with.

Males also continue to dominate the culinary world because of the attitude of French chefs that has carried over to the United States. There were French chefs who even refused to allow a woman in their kitchens. Even though this attitude is changing, women can still be made to feel unfit for their position. Men have preconceived notions that women are incapable of doing the job because it involves physical strength. But it doesn't take brawn to lift a pot. It takes brains, a partner, and a pivot.

At times, kitchens are not easy places for women to survive in because men don't want to make it easy for them to be there. There are huge male egos to deal with and creative personalities. Sara has worked for 7 years in a number of atmospheres. She has worked with all male staffs, all female staffs, and with a complement of both. She believes that a blend of men and women usually works best.

Women chefs are usually more even-tempered than are male chefs. Women typically handle stress in the kitchen in a way that should be modeled by men. When there is a rush and a waitstaff person returns a rack of lamb to be cooked more, a woman on the broiler station would say "OK," put it in the broiler, and when she thought it was done, would turn around and hand it to the waitstaff person. Male chefs, on the other hand, commonly throw a temper tantrum, toss the lamb on the grill, burn it to a crisp, let it cool, and then hand it back to the waitstaff person.

Another reason that there are fewer women, Sara believes, is that women experience a conflict between responsibilities to family and career. Although she thinks of herself as a feminist to the core, she states that once her children were born she felt that they needed a mother and wanted to be there for them whenever possible. Restaurant work hours of 60 to 70 hours do not lend themselves to allowing for much time with family. Chef Moulton cannot miss the school play and does not send her children off without the brownies for their birthday party.

The husband of Jody Adams (a chef at the Rialto in Boston) truly does the major "kid duty," Sara tells us. A former boss at *Gourmet Magazine* also had a husband who quit his construction job to stay at home with the children. But finding a man who is willing to work full-time in the home is not always possible, especially when finances depend on a single income.

Regardless of gender, it is difficult for individuals to make money even as a big executive chef. Most money is made from high volume catering or in high-volume restaurants. When individuals enter the food industry, there's usually more of an artistic attraction than a monetary lure. But, regardless of the salary, a chef will always be able to put some food on the table. The lack of health benefits and retirement are also important considerations for women.

Mentoring and Awareness

In 1982, Sara Moulton co-founded the New York Women's Culinary Alliance in an effort to bring women together to network. Today the Alliance is made up of over 200 women members. The by-laws require that members attend at least four sponsored programs each month, or that they serve on a committee, or put on a program. A monthly newsletter and a job exchange network are also in place for members. Professional organizations such as this one provide women the opportunity to share ideas.

Influences

Sara Moulton credits M.F.K. Fisher's books about food in part for influencing her interest in cuisine. Women chefs who have influenced Sara's career, include Julia Child and Lydia Shire. Julia Child, whom she had the opportunity to work with, encouraged her to get going, and to "get this job and that job." Julia helped her to secure an apprenticeship in France as well. Lydia Shire set a good example for Sara to model her career.

Although cooking began as a past time, Sara's interest in this career grew in time and with her mother's prodding. She had gone to college and had earned an undergraduate degree. After college she was floundering as a cook in a bar, when her mom wrote to Julia Child and to Craig Clairborne to ask what her daughter had to do to become a chef? Craig Clairborne answered that "She should go to cooking school; she should go to the Culinary Institute of America." So she did…and the rest is history.

You'll need to remind yourself frequently that you're a worthy human being, because there will be people in your path who'll make it their business to tear you down (and especially if you're a woman, you may want to do it yourself).

Maria Shriver, **Ten Things I Wish I'd known— Before I Went Out Into the Real World**

CASE DISCUSSION

Chef Moulton has given us a great perspective on how many women in industry feel today. We are grateful for her willingness to speak out on this role. Working through the questions that follow may help you to uncover some unknown biases.

CASE QUESTIONS

1. Are you surprised that women often experience the kitchen in this way?

2. What beliefs and attitudes must change for women to feel more welcomed in the food industry?

3. How many famous female chefs can you name?

4. What is your perspective on women in the kitchen?

Sara Moulton is Executive Chef at Gourmet Magazine, Host of Food Network's "Cooking Live", Host of Food Network's "Sara's Secrets", and Food Editor for "Good Morning America"

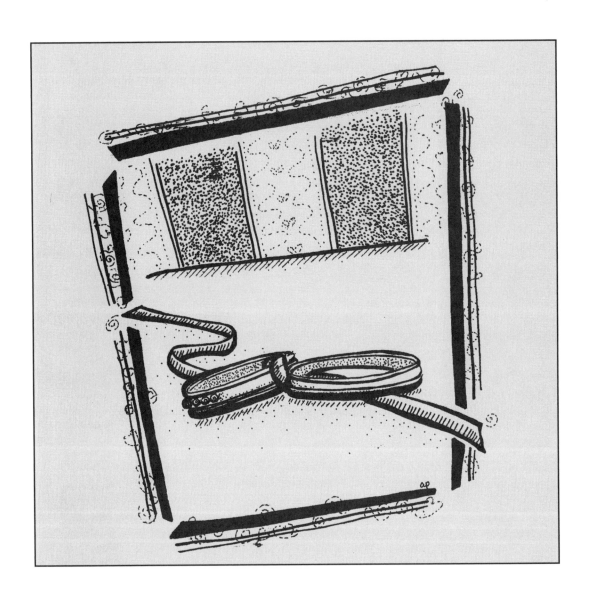

Can Chefs Have a Healthy Personal Life?

Seduced by Success

I began in the food business as a young man. I had no idea what to expect. I knew I loved to cook, and I knew that I was willing to work hard at it. I was young, and I believed in myself. So how did I become someone who gave in to temptation?

Camera, Action, Lights, Temptation

How does often unsolicited fame happen to chefs? Chefs literally appear to generate a masterpiece within a matter of minutes. They create works of art that appeal to the eyes, the palate, and the sense of smell. They are admired for their skills and they seem to emanate a sense of perfection that many find irresistible. People love to hob-knob with well-known chefs, and chefs come to love the attention. Exposure to constant flattery leads to inflated egos, a feeling of invincibility, and a vulnerability to temptation.

When a chef's career becomes his/her life and his/her identity, it is inevitable that his/her family life will be impacted negatively. Success requires dedication and long hours of work—sometimes 80 hours per week. There are business partners to deal with, investors to please, and customers to satisfy.

It Doesn't Mean Anything

For some men it may be easy to separate love and sex. For others, this is not so easy. I become involved in illicit relationships to escape work pressures. Sex outside of marriage provides me with ego gratification. Opportunities are common, and I find myself not refusing these advances. I look for reasons for my behavior and seem not to find any. With restaurants to run, cookbooks to write, menus to create, and employees to care for, I feel stressed. The long hours away from home, and an ego that loves constant stroking lead me to turn to sex outside of marriage. I never plan to be unfaithful to my wife or to jeopardize my marriage. I love my wife. Every time I'm unfaithful I'm disappointed with myself, and I try to convince myself that it won't happen again. I know that I would never be where I am today without my wife's support, and I know that I'm lucky that she stays with me.

From the Wife's Perspective

My husband's unfaithfulness hurts me. How can he give in to temptation? I don't separate sex from love and I don't understand how he does what he does. Career is important, but so is family. I find it embarrassing to think that others would think that I might not be able to satisfy his needs. Living with his infidelity hurts me every day. Intellectually, I know that the choices he makes have to do with the pressures caused by long hours and the attention he receives as a chef. But I doubt his love, and I feel vulnerable. I wish I could say that I don't worry that it will ever happen again. Unfortunately, it takes years to rebuild trust. The temptation is probably never going to go away. Even though I don't think that his deeds are the result of negative feelings toward me, I constantly worry about the attractive women at work.

It is Easier to be at Work

It is easy in the restaurant business to get caught up in gratification. Listening to customers' praises and having a glass of champagne at the end of the evening is part of the glamour of the restaurant industry. The idea of going home at night often pales in comparison to that. Maybe the house isn't air-conditioned and it's 90 degrees out, one of the kids is sick, or your spouse wasn't in the best of moods when you left in the morning.

Staying at home is not always an easy thing to do. I love being a mother and working part time. I would not trade that experience for anything. However, when my husband comes home and says that he's tired, I feel the same way. I guess that maybe I too am looking for some recognition for what I contribute. At work my husband is applauded and cheered for his presentations. When he acts as a husband and father, there is no applause. Even though we love him deeply and want him to be a part of us, we figure that it is his job and his responsibility to be a husband and father.

A Love Story, Warts and All

The weird thing is that except for this one flaw, he is a terrific guy. When we are together we are just that. We have a great time, and we communicate well. I can ask him anything, and he will tell me the truth no matter how difficult or painful it is. Would we like it to "go away?" I think that he would like it to disappear, possibly more than I would. He doesn't want to hurt me, but I know he is not able to stop himself from having these affairs. In a way I understand his battle. I am overweight, and I can't tell you how many times that I've promised myself that I would go on a diet, and then I fail again. Although both these problems might seem simple, neither really is. Each of us is a collection of past experiences. Our past plays a role in our present. Leaving would be an easy decision if I did not feel there were so many other good things about our relationship. Leaving him also goes against my sense of responsibility to family

I don't want to hear any more about being sorry. I will always love my husband, but I feel like a babysitter. My vows were for better or worse, and we are trying to make something worse better. Despite all the pain and hurt, we have good moments in our marriage. We have fun together, and most importantly we share a history. We have had some terrible times, and some wonderful times together. What would leaving prove? Anybody can give up.

It is easy to leave when there is hurt. For a long time I was deeply sad about my marriage, but somehow we survived. I know that he wants to stop what he does—he struggles with his decisions. For now, the hurt is not enough to drown our marriage—there are too many other good things about our family life and relationship that outweigh this pain. We must continue to face these issues together.

Forgiveness is a choice, always a choice. It is not a forced requirement.

Michele Weldon, **I Closed My Eyes**

CASE DISCUSSION

This couple shows courage in addressing an issue that chefs might face. Although this topic is a difficult one to discuss, doing so may prevent other families from such a tragedy. The following questions are directed at addressing the stressful life of a chef.

CASE QUESTIONS

1. Given the pressures that chefs face, how can they maintain strong ethical values?

2. What can chefs do to protect against becoming victims of flattery and fame?

3. How can chefs maintain a good family life?

4. What advice can you give this couple to help resolve their issues?

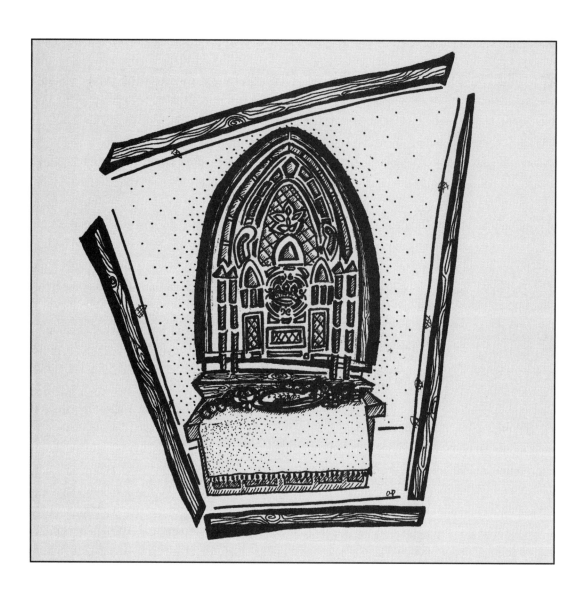

An Inside Look at Charlie Trotter's

The Front of the House and the Back of the House Issue

We called Charlie Trotter to help us answer a frequently asked question: How is it that in his restaurant the people in the front of the house actually get along with those in the back of the house? Charlie said that it is easy. We contend that if it were easy, more people would be doing it. Charlie then invited us to visit his property to see for ourselves.

Inside the Organization

Every evening at Charlie Trotter's restaurant begins with a staff meeting. There is no joking around or lack of attention when this takes place. People at Charlie's accept the business of hospitality seriously. His employees know that their mission is to do anything possible to make guests feel comfortable. But there is more to it than just that. Beneath the words and the service there is an elegance and civility that is rather unique in this culture. Daily staff meetings take place in one of the kitchens. Employees wait for Charlie's opening words before any conversation takes place. He simply asks: "What have you got?" To this question, individuals respond with a number of comments or questions. People speak on a variety of topics: "Would Charlie come to a particular guest's table? Are we going to expand in London?" etc.

Charlie has three points that serve as underlying principles that contribute to the secret of his success in getting the front of the house employees to get along with the back of the house. Every employee is paid on a salary basis; each employee is cross-trained; and all workers clean the restaurant each night after closing. It's that simple! And it works!

Everyone is on Salary?

Both front-of-the house and back-of-the house employees are salaried. Why? Because they are valued as employees. A "back waiter" who has worked at the restaurant for eight years will earn more than a back waiter's pay because of his loyalty to the organization. Employees do not know what other workers earn. Salaries are kept confidential among three parties: the individual, Charlie, and the bookkeeper. Tips go into a general pool. The waitstaff work in cooperation with chefs because their focus is not on their individual tip revenue. Employees say the money is fair. Employees at Charlie's have excellent medical and dental plans; they are treated as professionals. "It all boils down to how you treat people," says Charlie.

Walking a Mile in Another's Shoes

Cross training, or walking a mile in another's shoes, is another innovative method for team building that Charlie uses. Pastry chefs, glass polishers, and waitstaff assume other roles if the situation dictates. Everyone has spent time in another person's shoes. If a job looks easy, it is only because it is executed with grace and skill. Cross-training saves money, and it eliminates unhealthy competition. This practice also alleviates boredom and complacency. Employees are on a rotation so that they are able to understand the demands of a variety of jobs. Trading places encourages individuals to learn more about the operation and to seek advancement when they feel that they are ready.

Equal Opportunity Cleaning

Chef Trotter insists that everyone help in cleaning the restaurant when the evening's service is completed. There is a shared experience of ownership when the cleaning is done by employees. There are no "prima donnas" at Charlie Trotter's. The task of cleaning is merely an extension of sharing jobs. Charlie's standards are high, and the property must meet these demands. Detail cleaning is performed by an outside cleaning service. To quote Charlie, "The way the dumpster looks is as important as how the front door looks."

Culture is Stronger Than Policy

Employees do not have a policy manual at Charlie Trotter's. Simply stated, the policy is summarized in the question that employees must repeatedly ask themselves when they perform their tasks, "Is it the best it can be for the guest?" The idea is to aim for excellence but to go beyond. No one stands around because there is always something to do. Individuals are assigned to a particular job, but if something needs to be done, whoever is available does it.

When people are exposed to a culture in which they are consistently required to learn, they continue to do so. Employees regularly learn from one another. They are humble in their roles and they receive plenty of feed-back about what is an acceptable standard. There is no boredom here; as soon as one task is mastered there is another skill to be acquired. There is always room to discover how to do something even better. While the organization is not compartmentalized, it is remarkably organized. People have places, jobs and roles.

We asked the employees what they thought of the whole rotation design, the salary idea, and clean-up duty. Many said that they thought the money was fair but weren't wild about the clean-up duties, but they all replied that they learned an awful lot every day. Employees experience job satisfaction and a deep sense of pride because they also feel a sense of accomplishment. They stay because they can later say that they worked at Charlie Trotter's, and this is an automatic ticket to wherever they may want to go. The culture is strong and impressive.

The Table in the Kitchen

The courtesy afforded others in the kitchen also surprised us. No obscenities were heard from across the line and individuals were not confrontational. The kitchen, like the front-of-the house reflected respect and dignity. The executive chef also let us in on a little secret— the table at the end of the room. In the back end of the kitchen there is a table set up where 6 restaurant guests may actually dine while having a bird's eye view of the kitchen, and the opportunity to hob-knob with the staff. Charlie also hosts a guest (who's not a chef) in the kitchen each night that is invited to cook on the line with the experts.

A State of the Art Kitchen With Visual Appeal

Sitting in the kitchen is quite nice. The kitchen range, complete with brass fittings was made in Lyon, France. There is a wood-fired grill, and copper pots with stainless linings that decorate the line and reflect off the brush aluminum ceilings. The glass cabinetry is both beautiful and practical as it allows chefs to see the utensils they need. There are no walk-ins, only reach-ins. The kitchen is impeccable even during peak hours. There is a *garde-manger* area where delights such as cucumber jelly and smoked salmon are prepared. The kitchen is actually rather small, but it is well organized and efficiently arranged.

The Cuisine is the Centerpiece

Everything in Charlie Trotter's restaurant contributes to enhancing the dining experience. There are no large fragrant flower bouquets to over power the aromatic flavors of the cuisine. The décor consists of modest pictures, mirrors, and plaques, and it is always the meal that is the centerpiece.

"I am in the business of growing people—people who are stronger, healthier, more autonomous, more self-reliant, and more competent."

Robert Greenleaf, **Servant Leadership**

CASE DISCUSSION

Charlie Trotter is a gracious man who knows that valuing employees pays big dividends. He understands the power of creating a culture that can keep his mission alive. His ideas are revolutionary and perhaps even a bit bold, but they do work.

CASE QUESTIONS

1. Is it possible that motivation decreases when all employees are salaried? Explain your answer.

2. Can American employees accept the team ideal even though their cultural socialization revolves around personal achievement? Explain.

3. How does an employer using this management model (one that does not use a policy manual) protect himself from potential lawsuits?

4. What is Charlie Trotter's most powerful leadership strategy?

Chef Charlie Trotter is the owner of Charlie Trotter's in Chicago

Part 2
Activities and Points to Ponder on Leadership, Management, and Organizational Theory

Activity# 16: Two Loves and a Wish

Getting Feedback from Those you Teach and Lead

An exercise that those in leadership roles perform in order to extract feedback from employees is known as *Two Loves and a Wish*. In this exercise the employer distributes index cards and asks employees to write two things that they love about the organization and one thing that they would change if they could. The exercise provides employees the opportunity to voice their opinions anonymously, and supplies employers with both positive and negative input.

Activity # 17: The Ingredients of Successful Change

To achieve successful change . . .

✔ Position a hero in charge of the process.

✔ Recognize a real threat from the outside.

✔ Make transition rituals the pivotal elements of change.

✔ Provide transition training in new values and behavior patterns.

✔ Bring in outside shamans.

✔ Build tangible symbols of the new directions.

✔ Insist on the importance of (job) security in transition.

How can an organization begin and continue this process?

From *Corporate Cultures: The Rites and Rituals of Corporate Life* by B. Chrisman, T.E. Deal, and A.A. Kennedy

Activity # 18 Bowen: Family Roles (the family as an emotional unit)

M. Bowen, developed a family systems theory that conceptualizes the family as an emotional unit, or a network of interlocking relationships. His theory is best understood when analyzed within a multigenerational or historical framework. Bowen's work makes a significant contribution to the way in which we understand roles and relationships. The presence of an alcoholic father, a rageaholic mother, or an anexoric teenager in a family structure uses up all the family resources, and becomes the center of the family dynamic. Others in the family may need to assume other roles represented around the circle in order to survive within this structure. This same theory can be applied to the organization. When an out of control employer monopolizes the circle, those around him/her will adapt to these roles, and the organization will become sick just as the family dynamic does. Bowen theorizes that the following outcomes will occur in an organization or a family system:

- ✔ triangulation (gossip)
- ✔ emotional cut-off (do not speak)
- ✔ enmeshment (too close; little autonomy)
- ✔ family projection process (working issues with children)
- ✔ multigenerational transmission (sins of the parent on the children)
- ✔ societal regression (messed up society)

"Family Roles" by M. Bowen (1979)

Questions

1. Based on Bowen's 6 Points, what are some steps that might be taken to improve an unhealthy organization?

2. What implications does the model have for impacting people's behavior in the workplace?

3. If you were to apply Bowen's six outcomes in light of your workplace, what would the results be?

4. How does this model increase your understanding of what may motivate the behavior of others?

5. How can you keep yourself emotionally healthy in an unhealthy organization?

Activity #19 Family Illness in Children

	Visible Qualities	Inner Feelings	Represents To Family
Family hero	Visible success Does what's right	Inadequate	Self-worth (family can be proud)
Scapegoat	Hostility Defiance Anger	Hurt Guilt	Takes focus off the alcoholic
Lost child	Withdrawn Loner	Loneliness Unimportant	Relief (one child not to worry about)
Mascot	Fragile Immature Needs protection	Fear	Fun and humor (comic relief)

Activity #19 continued

	Characteristics	Possible Future Characteristics	
		Without Help	With Help
Family hero	High-achiever Grades, friends, sports	Workaholic Never wrong Responsible for everything Marry dependant	Accepts failure Responsible for self, not all Good executives
Scapegoat	Negative attention Won't compete with family hero	Unplanned pregnancy Trouble maker in school and later in office Prison	Accepts responsibility Good counselors Courage Ability to see reality
Lost Child	Invisible Quiet No friends Follower Trouble making decisions	Little zest for life Sexual identity problems Promiscuous or stays alone often dies at an early age	Independent Talented Creative Imaginative Self-actualized
Mascot	Hyperactive Learning disabilities Short attention span	Ulcers Can't handle stress Compulsive clown marry hero for care Remains immature	Takes care of self No longer clown Fun to be with Good sense of humor

Colman, H. *The Family Trap.*
Model designed by Linda Mix and adapted from *The Family Trap*.

Using this chart, evaluate your current business.

Activity # 20: How to be an Optimist

The pessimist believes bad events stem from permanent conditions	The optimist finds the inaccuracies
The pessimist allows a disappointment in one area of his/her life to pervade the rest	The optimist limits the influence of the event on his/her life
When things go wrong, the pessimist blames herself/ himself even if it wasn't all her/his fault	The optimist doesn't always blame herself/himself
The pessimist catastrophizes	The optimist looks for a solution

In which column do you find yourself most often? Why? What would you need to do to move to the optimist's column, if you are not already there?

Adapted from *Good Housekeeping* by T. Eberlin and *Learned Optimism* by M. Seligman

Activity # 21 Effective Leadership

A boss drives. A leader leads.

A boss relies on authority. A leader relies on cooperation.

A boss says "I." A leader says "We."

A boss creates fear. A leader creates confidence.

A boss knows how. A leader shows how.

A boss creates resentment. A leader breads enthusiasm.

How could you change your workplace to fit Glasser's model?

Glasser, W. *The Quality School: Managing Students Without Coercion*.

Activity # 22: On Being a Synergistic Leader

Identification

How do (1) you like to work in a group?

What was (my) your greatest accomplishment by (my) yourself and as a member of a group?

If (I) you don't agree with a suggested idea, person, or thing, what do (I) you do?

Inclusion

Who are we as a group?

Can we meet without all of us being here?

When a discussion becomes difficult do we wish certain persons were not in the group?

Acceptance

When we're together, we can do anything.

This group can produce under any conditions.

There is no question that this group is producing more than any of us would have imagined in the beginning.

Dependence

When will we meet and for how long?

Will we adjourn if we find that we are not being very productive?

How often do we need to meet to keep our group in a supportive working mode?

Fusion

Who completed that job?

How much did a certain individual do?

Where did we get that suggestion?

Affirmation

Our synergistic energy will cause us to produce more than we ever anticipated.

Our energy from the synergy of each one of us and our group will overcome fatigue and make us more productive.

Our group will sustain all threats of external dissociation by knowing that our power of synergy will add to our energy and purpose.

Confirmation

Are there any doubts that we can do the work?

What outside factors might prevent us from accomplishing our tasks?

If we are challenged as to our ability to perform by an outside authority, what would be our action and reaction?

How might leaders use this model to evaluate group dynamics?

Wolfe, R. *Synergy: Increasing Productivity with People, Ideas, and Things*

Activity # 23: One-Minute Reprimand Exercise

1. Tell people beforehand that you are going to let them know how they are doing.

2. Reprimand people immediately.

3. Tell people what they did wrong (be specific).

4. Tell people how you feel about what they did wrong in no uncertain terms.

5. Stop for a few seconds of uncomfortable silence to let them *feel* how you feel.

6. Shake hands or touch them in a way that lets them know that you are honestly on their side.

7. Remind them of how much you value them.

8. Reaffirm that you think well of them but not of their performance in this situation.

9. Realize that when the reprimand is over, it's over.

From *The One-Minute Manager* by K. Blanchard, and S. Johnson

Activity # 24: One-Minute Praising Exercise

1. Tell people up front that you are going to let them know how they are doing.

2. Praise people immediately.

3. Tell people what they did right (be specific).

4. Tell people how good you feel about what they did right, and how it helps the organization and the other people who work there.

5. Stop for a moment of silence to let them *feel* how good you feel.

6. Encourage them to do more of the same.

7. Shake hands or touch them in a way that makes it clear that you support their success in the organization.

From *The One-Minute Manager* by K. Blanchard, and S. Johnson

Activity # 25: Refusal Skills Exercise

1. Identify the behavior in which the person is asking you to be involved.

2. Offer an alternate plan and invite them to participate in your plan.

3. If they refuse, politely decline participation in the activity.

Natural Helpers— Refusal Skills

Points to Ponder # 26: Steps in Managing Angry People

Ask the question "Am I dealing with focused or non-focused anger?"

Focused Anger—focused on a person, thing or event
Task = interrupt the anger

Non-Focused Anger—unfocused on any specific person, thing, or event
Task = use supervisory role

3 Steps in Anger Intervention

1. Know your task = Break the chain link by link— interrupt the anger— acknowledge
   Don't say: "Calm down" or "I understand"

2. Bridge to content (not feelings)

3. Paraphrase—summarize with intensity

3 Areas That Have to be Managed

1. Know your task (diffuse)

2. Get emotional control of yourself

3. Use Bias Management (body language)

Adapted from lectures given by Hatch, J. *Steps in Managing Angry People*

Activity #27: Rules for open Communication

1. Both parties state their problem
   ✔ Use "I" statements
   ✔ Indicate a willingness to help resolve the problem
   ✔ Stay in the present and the future
   ✔ Stick to the topic at hand
   ✔ Ask for specific changes

2. Hear them out
   ✔ Don't interrupt
   ✔ Acknowledge their viewpoint
   ✔ Restate what you've heard
   ✔ Offer an apology if appropriate
   ✔ Ask clarifying questions
   ✔ Stay in the present and the future

3. Look for areas of agreement
   ✔ Point out general interests that you have in common
   ✔ Make a positive and optimistic statement

4. Request behavior changes only
   ✔ Think "power with" rather than "power over"— this will guarantee that your attitude will be one that invites resolution.
   ✔ Realize that what's happening now isn't meeting your interests. It's worth trying try something new.
   ✔ Plan your discussion, especially your opening.
   ✔ Keep your goal in mind. Have notes on hand, if needed

From *Conflict Resolution and Confrontation Skills* by H. Rhode in Career Track

Activity # 28: Discussion Questions for Decision-Making within an Organization

1. How did things get this way?

2. Who are the key players in the organization?

3. Who stands to be impacted by change?

4. What are the possible applications for this decision?

5. What role does such a decision play in the humanity of the organization?

6. What can be done to change the situation?

7. What happens if this situation continues?

8. Is this a universal problem in our industry? Why or why not?

9. What is the moral issue?

10. Can this event be compared with any other in the history of the organization?

Activity # 29 Elements of Cultures

✔ Specific language

✔ Artifacts

✔ Symbols

✔ Rituals and ceremonies

✔ Myths and stories

✔ Norms

✔ Roles

✔ Specific values (beliefs, attitudes, shared meanings)

What would it take to change these elements of culture in a work place?

Activity # 30 The Leadership Challenge for Employers and Employees

Develop a team activity that can demonstrate these five pivotal organizational components.

- ✔ challenge the process
- ✔ inspire a shared vision
- ✔ enable others to act
- ✔ model the way
- ✔ encourage the heart

From *The Leadership Challenge: How to Keep Getting Extraordinary Things Done in Organizations* by J. Kouzes, and B. Posner

Part 2
Books for Further Reading on Leadership, Management, and Organizational Theory

References

Blanchard, K., W. Oncken, and H. Burrows. *The One Minute Manager Meets the Monkey.* New York: Quill William Morrow, 1989.

Brim, O. and S. Wheeler. *Socialization Through the Life Cycle.* New York: John Wiley and Sons, Inc. , 1996.

Clarke, P. *Lessons in Excellence from Charlie Trotter.* California: Ten Speed Press, 1999.

Colman, H. *The Family Trap.* New York: William Morrow and Company Publishers, 1982.

Ehrenreich, B. *The Fear of Falling.* New York: Harper Perennial, 1990.

Gardner, J. *On Leadership.* New York: The Free Press, 1990.

Greenleaf, R. *Servant Leadership.* New Jersey: Paulist Press, 1977.

Johnson, S. *Who Moved My Cheese?* New York: G.P. Putnam's Sons, 1998.

Johnson, S. and K. Blanchard. *The One-Minute Manager.* Berkley Publishing Group, 1993.

King, M., Jr. *The Strength to Love.* Philadelphia: Fortress Press, 1963.

King, M., Jr. *The Measure of A Man.* Philadelphia: Fortress Press, 1998.

Kouzes, J. and B. Posner. *The Leadership Challenge: How to keep getting extraordinary things done in organizations.* Jossey-Bass Management Series, 1996.

Markham, D. *Spiritlinking Leadership.* New Jersey: Paulist Press, 1999.

McCall, N. *Makes Me Wanna Holler: A young black man in America.* New York: Vintage Books, 1994.

Phillips, D. *Lincoln on Leadership.* New York: Warner Books, 1992.

Rifkin, J. *The End of Work.* New York: G.P. Putnam's Sons, 1995.

Raelin, J. *Clash of Cultures.* Boston: Harvard Business School Press, 1985.

Senge, P. *The Fifth Discipline.* New York: Doubleday, 1990.

Shriver, M. *Ten Things I Wish I'd Known.* New York: Warner Books, 2000.

Weldon, M. *I Closed My Eyes.* Minnesota: Hazeldon Information and Educational Services, 1999

Wegscheider, S. *The Family Trap.* Johnson Institute, 1976.

Wolfe, R. *Synergy.* Iowa: Kendall/Hunt Publishing Company, 1993.

Journal Articles and Studies for Further Reading on Leadership, Management, and Organizational Theory

Gouldner, A. " Cosmopolitans and Locals: Toward an analysis of latent social roles." Administrative Science Quarterly, 1957.

Gundry, L. & Rosseau, D. (1994). "Critical incidents in communicating culture to newcomers: The meaning is the message." *Human Relations*, 47(9) (1994): 1063-1069.

Hatch, J. "Dealing with angry kids." Adapted from lectures (1996).

Louis, M. (1980). "Surprise and sense making: What newcomers experience in entering unfamiliar organizational settings." *Administrative Quarterly*, 25 (1980): 230-231.

Van Maanen, J. & Schein, E. (1979). " Toward a theory of organizational socialization." *Research in Organizational Behavior*, 1 (1979): 210-214.